Cancer Disarmed

Expanded Version

Healing Benefits of Fermented and Nitrogenated Soy

By
Nina Anderson, S.P.N.
in cooperation with Dr. Howard Peiper

Published by
Safe Goods Publishing

Cancer Disarmed
Expanded Version

ISBN 1-884820-73-5
978-1884820-73-5
Library of Congress Catalog Card Number 2002096385
Printed in USA

Cancer Disarmed is not intended as medical advice, but as suggested
complementary therapeutic regimens, to be considered only if deemed
adequate by both patients and their chosen health professional. It is written solely for informational and educational purposes.

Safe Goods Publishing
561 Shunpike Rd.
Sheffield, MA 01257
413-229-7935

FOREWORD

"Hundreds of millions of dollars are spent annually on new and improved chemicals that prove or confirm that they can kill mutated (cancer) cells. However, they also destroy the host cells. *Cancer Disarmed* is well organized, and reveals a totally nontoxic companion to the currently accepted "gold-standard" for treatments of neoplastic disease. Ms. Anderson does a scholarly job of revealing the potency of this incredible ancient soy food supplement. The soy beverage described within, has built-in isoflavones, hyper activated by fermentation, which in turn changes not only our T cells, but directs the built-in nitrogen into the mutated cells, thus converting to nitric acid and killing them.

I have had the privilege of being the husband of a cancer survivor and observing firsthand, the incredible immune-boosting properties of the liquid soybean phytochemical beverage. After some very unprofessional surgical and oncological consultations, my wife opted to go exclusively with the fermented soy, prayer, body-balance, and exercise. I am happy to report that three years have gone by and she is well.

This book is not intended to be a substitute for seeking medical advice, but as a resource for you to be enabled as a well-informed participant in the successful physician to patient team."

-William J. Saccoman, M.D.
Charter Fellow of American Academy of Family Physicians since 1973; Diploma–American College for Advancement in Medicine.

INTRODUCTION

Over the years I have become interested specifically in the advantages of the more digestible versions (fermented) of this beneficial soy. The medicinal power of the soy supplementation process derives its effect from the process of reducing the constituents into a small form that can easily enter a cell. Having known of the benefits of tiny crystalloid mineral molecules that can easily penetrate cells to improve cellular function, I learned of a soy product with similar attributes.

My interest in nutritional disease-fighting properties always left me in a state of consternation over the many types of cancers and their lethal power. Through my studies of this new soy therapy, I found it exciting to understand how a cancer cell works, and what can be used to undermine its deadly assignment. The disarming of cancer cells through nitrogenation of a soy phytochemical supplement has treatment promise on a wide scale. It is a real advance in adjuvant (helping) cancer therapy; one that cannot be ignored. To help with understanding how disease impacts the body, I have used several informational platforms, including a presentation of the immune system fighting an intergalactic conflict.

The soy therapy outlined to disarm cancer cells does not exclude current medical treatments, such as chemotherapy and radiation. Nor is the immune system ignored in the battle to minimize and dispose cancer cells. This soy-therapy approach may give you a new perspective, even when used as treatment for what are regarded as the "low survival" cancers. The research studies I was privileged to review are from respected medical sources, primarily conducted in China. The testimonials we reveal are true and accountable. The majority of these survivors have medical file documentation, with backup from attending, licensed physicians to attest to their stories. I hope you will share this information with your friends and family.

-Nina Anderson,
ISSA-certified Specialist in Performance Nutrition

TABLE OF CONTENTS

1

CANCER: *The battle waged inside your body*

For a moment, let's visualize we are in the twenty first century, battling aliens to keep our human species alive. Our planet has undergone changes that have resulted in weakened defenses. Alien forces infiltrating our colony are already hiding inside our fortress. The aliens' plan to defeat us includes reducing our core food supply, and mating with humans.

Over time, the hybrid offspring react like aliens. Aliens have a direct link to our food chain, so they get the choice vitamin-rich entrees, and leave us with the garbage. These intruders also have learned which type of weapons can kill them, and have removed from our planet the necessary materials required to create these weapons. We no longer have the ability to destroy the aliens, because we are living off insufficiently fortified food, and our children have turned against us. What hope do we have for survival? If only a "superhero" could alter the alien's thought processes enough to cut off their food pillaging, and allow us to gather the materials to build our weapons again, so we can destroy them once and for all.

What happens inside our bodies when cancer cells start replicating unchecked is exactly identical to the "aliens" of our tale. Our immune system is a strategic defense system that automatically knows what to do when a foreign intruder threatens our health. Cancer cells live harmlessly in the body as long as the immune system is operating properly. T cells act as the avengers, converting nitrogen into nitric acid that they then release onto the cancer cells, dissolving them. Normal cells are protected from this defensive assault by a coating of the enzyme superoxide dismutase (SOD).[1] This

---

[1] To maintain adequate levels of SOD, it is important to keep a strong balance of electrolyte minerals, specifically manganese and selenium, which stimulate the body's production of SOD.

coating is absent in cancer cells. Cancer cells seek out the nitrogen in our body's protein, thus depleting the nitrogen that the T cells need for the production of their "assault weapon." Nitrogen comes from protein stored in the muscle tissue, and is a target for the cancer cell. The breakdown of muscle in cancer patients, cachexia (the medical term) is a condition generally referred to as the "wasting disease." It literally causes weight loss and muscle protein loss, general debility and lack of appetite, all factors that severely compromise the health of the patient. It is estimated that up to 40 percent of all cancer patients die from malnutrition, not from the cancer.[2] Without a nitrogen source to produce the nitric acid, the T cells technically run out of "ammunition."

Cancer cells are quite proficient at reproduction and task-control of the cells. Normal cells are programmed to die at a normal rate, after producing daughter cells that resemble themselves. Cancer cells alter the programming so they don't die, and their daughter cells are reprogrammed to live longer. This creates a mass of dysfunctional cells, which is what is commonly called a tumor. To thrive and grow, these cells need to be fed. They draw nutrients from an in-growth of blood capillaries that feed them. To further defend itself from the immune system that may try to cut off its blood (food) supply, the cancer cell grows a tough protein coating that is thirteen times thicker than a normal cell. When there are many cancer cells, they can circulate through the blood to other parts of the body, called metastasizing.

You can now begin to understand just how well programmed cancer cells are. The immune system has a tough job to do, and needs support. Research points to three main causes—and most probably a combination of them: poor nutrition; mental and emotional stress; and toxins in foods, cosmetics, household cleaners, lawn treatments, etc. The first thing we must do is to boost our immune system. We can begin by restoring our mineral balance through

---

[2] Grant, J.P., "Proper use and recognized role of total parenteral nutrition in the cancer patient," *Nutrition,* vol.6, no.4, July/Aug, 1990.

electrolyte supplementation, and increasing the assimilation of food nutrients by adding digestive enzymes to our meals (Refer to the next chapter). Also, adding antioxidant foods or antioxidant supplements to our body can build up our reserves of free-radical fighters.

At least 40 percent of those who die with cancer, do so because of protein calorie malnutrition, not cancer, according to Patrick Quillian, Ph.D., R.D., C.N.S.[3] Ross Pelton, Ph.D., who was the administrator at Hospital Santa Monica, treated cancer patients who had cachexia. After administering a protocol of a fermented soy beverage, the patients experienced an increase in energy levels and regained their appetites. He attributes their improvement to the high protein content of the soy as well as its anticancer agents. A mature soybean is approximately 42 percent protein and actually contains more protein than any other plant. It is a "complete protein," since it provides essential amino acids.[4] Once the patients regained strength, they were able to continue the alternative and complementary cancer treatment protocols.

Eating specific formulations of soy can provide cancer-fighting compounds, called phytochemicals. In order for these phytochemicals to do their job and cause the cancer to self-destruct, they must get into the cell. When soy proteins have been *fermented* and *nitrogenated,* they become hydrolysed into bioactive amino acids. These acids, being small molecules, are better able to permeate the cell wall, and are helped to do so by the fact that cancer cells foraging for nitrogen will absorb the nitrogenised bioactive amino acids. These carry with them undetected, immune-supporting compounds consisting of isoflavones, protease inhibitors, saponins, phytosterols, and phytic acids, which all have anticancer properties. Of these compounds, the isoflavones *genistein* and *daidzein,* and their metabolites, individually have the most powerful anticancer effects.

---

[3] Quillian, Patrick, Ph.D., R.D., C.N.S., *Beating Cancer with Nutrition,* 1994.
[4] Colebank, Susan, "Deconstructing Soy," *Health Supplement Retailer,* April 2002.

However, collectively the other anticancer compounds in soy produce greater cancer cell deaths than the isoflavones do as a class. Once inside the cell they cause cancer cells to re-differentiate and revert to normal cells, which in turn restores their programmed cell death resulting in their death (apoptosis) as they would during their normal cycle. Also slowed, and eventually inhibited, is the in-growth of capillaries, thereby effectively cutting off the cancer cell's food supply (neo-angiogenesis). The immune system can then do its job of disabling and removing cancerous growth.

The isoflavones *genistein* and *daidzein,* have the most powerful anticancer effects of all the phytochemicals in soy. Once inside the cell, they cause cancer to differentiate, and change back to normal cells, where they are reprogrammed to die, as they would in their normal cycle. Also slowed, and eventually inhibited, is the in-growth of blood capillaries, effectively cutting off the cancer cell's food supply. Not all forms of soy have the ability to penetrate the cancer cell wall. A specific process is necessary to reduce the phytochemical molecules to a miniscule size, for easy cell penetration. Also, the nitrogenation is essential to facilitate the uptake of the anticancer components by the nitrogen-seeking cancer cell. Manufacturers who extract single soybean components, such as soy protein or isoflavones may not be providing other beneficial nutrients that contribute to health. Soy as a food with all the nutrients intact is preferred to gain the maximum benefit. In the next several chapters, we will elaborate on the importance of maintaining the building blocks of our immune system, and how beneficial soy is in fighting cancer.

2

Immune Support

The entire body must be considered in order to reap maximum treatment results. The expression, "survival of the fittest," aptly applies to illness. Those of us who jeopardize our health by excessive smoking, drinking, poor diet, and lack of exercise are easy targets for disease. People who support their immune systems through proper preventive care seem to fare better when faced with viral attacks, chronic illness, and cancer. Statistics support this.

Many books have been written on cancer cures, and most of the nondrug recommendations focus on dietary regimens and supplementation with herbs, vitamins, or other nutrients. For many people, these suggestions are part of an overall treatment plan. But, why wait to get sick to address your health issues?

Several simple steps can be taken that are known to fortify your immune system. The most important is to re-mineralize your body. Depletion of minerals can be a result of modern farming methods, and the filtering of our water supplies. This results in the population at large experiencing a dearth of mineral-deficiency diseases. Researchers have found for example, the nutritional content of soybeans has varied up to 50 percent, depending on the minerals in the soil where they are grown. These and all other soil-grown foods may be lacking the very essential micronutrients that contribute to the cellular support necessary for optimum health.

The water we drink can also be hazardous to our health. Tap water, in most cases, should be purified either with a whole house filter or point-of-use unit at the faucet. Submicron ceramic filters can remove harmful bacteria and other contaminants, but systems such as reverse osmosis or distillation that are successful at eliminating a larger percentage of contaminants, also eliminate beneficial minerals from the water. Bottled water has most likely been run through one of these purification processes and may also be devoid of minerals. For cancer prevention and treatment it is essential to drink purified water. Putting the minerals back into the water is a necessity. This can be accomplished either by adding crystalloid liquid minerals to the water or taking an ionic supplement. Crystalloid and ionic are the smallest forms of a mineral molecule, and have greater success in permeating the cell wall. Minerals are intended to do their best work inside the cell. If the molecule is too large (such as a colloidal form), it will just float by the cell, with most of it either being excreted, or being tucked away in the joints for "later use," which can result in arthritic-like pain from excessive buildup.

Minerals are the basis for building a strong immune system. They facilitate communication within the body, and are the building blocks for all bodily functions. To be mineral deficient, is to put yourself at risk. Electrolyte minerals also raise oxygen levels. Cancer does not thrive in an oxygen-rich environment, so the addition of electrolytes is a strong preventive measure that we can maintain on a daily basis.

Another important factor in building and maintaining a strong immune system is the bioavailability (absorption and nutrient release) of the foods we eat. Soy has been called a "miracle" food, but like other beans and nuts which have a tough coating, untreated soy is difficult to digest. The healthy isoflavones in soy naturally consist of large molecular clusters that are hard for the digestive system to cleave and use. Babies who are given soy formula often cry afterwards as a result of gas buildup from trying to digest the soymilk, which just doesn't break down easily.

When we eat cooked or processed food, the natural digestive enzymes in the foods are killed by the high cooking temperature. Our pancreas produces enzymes to break down this food, but overuse due to a diet mainly of cooked foods, wears it out. We then digest less and less of our food, produce more stomach gas, have fermented (smelly) stools, and receive minimal nutrition from what we eat. This eating pattern does not aid the immune system. Just like your car won't run on gas that has water in it, our body is less efficient when most of the nutrients are not absorbed.

To facilitate better assimilation, we should consider adding digestive enzymes to our diet whenever we eat cooked food. This not only relieves stress on the pancreas, but, prevents the antioxidant enzymes from being solicited to digest a meal, when they should be out fighting free-radicals (oxidizing agents that damage healthy cells). It is suspected that soy, which is difficult to digest, can be broken down with supplemental enzymes, thereby releasing its beneficial nutrients.

If enzymes are in short supply, the body calls in the minerals to interact with the undigested food and carry it out of the body (chelation). When minerals are in short supply, problems may begin when they are solicited to join forces for tasking assignments; for example, in mineral dependent areas of the body, such as the brain. Extended mineral-deficient periods can affect organ function.

To protect your immune system, and support your pancreas (reducing stomachaches and, hopefully the need for antacids), supplement your diet with digestive enzymes. Enzymes facilitate absorption of nutrients. In your body, they set off a long list of chemical reactions necessary for cellular tasking of proper bodily function. Cancer cells only grow in an enzyme-deficient environment. Where enzymes are abundant, they wage war on cancer cells, identifying them as intruders and eradicating them. A lack of sufficient supply of enzymes will reduce this protection. Enzymes also break up cancer-causing waste in the body, removing it before it has a chance to develop into a hazardous mass.

Some studies have found that the enzyme Protease dissolves the protective, fibrous coating around cancer cells, making them more accessible to the immune system's "swat team." Protease also has been shown to help shrink tumors by removing abnormal tissue, and enhancing healthy tissue growth. Preventing cancer, therefore, starts with keeping the 'host' healthy, with minerals and enzymes forming the foundation for successful outcomes.

Dietary Recommendations:

- Alternate between raw foods and cooked foods meals
- Include a daily meal of fruit only (preferably in the morning): grapes (with seeds and skins), papaya, oranges, apple
- Daily serving of soup (primarily vegetables)
- Daily serving of cooked or raw vegetables: broccoli, carrots, celery, onions, green cabbage, red beet, parsley, garlic
- Starch: rice (preferable integral and as a whole meal, sweet corn
- Daily serving of nuts: almonds, walnuts
- Yogurt with friendly bifidius bacterial for colon health
- Fermented soya
- Oil: olive (cold pressed)
- Flesh foods: Fish, turkey
- Drinks: water, carrot juice (alone or with celery), beetroot, raw garlic, orange juice, lemon juice, green tea, parsley tea.

Foods to Avoid: sugar, artificial sweeteners, red meat and animal fats, fried food, tobacco, alcohol, refined flour (white bread), foods containing hydrogenated or partially-hydrogenated oil, caffeine

Supplements: Vitamin C, E, multi-vitamin, ionic minerals, essential fatty acids, antioxidant such as Rhodiola rosea, digestive enzymes, fermented soya

3

In Favor of Soy for Breast Cancer

The subject of "estrogen positive" breast cancers and the use of soy is one that has confused many women and is addressed in this chapter to clarify the issue.

The proper term is "estrogen *receptor* positive" breast cancer not "estrogen positive" as it is commonly stated. This term refers to breast cancer cells whose growth is *enhanced* by estrogen.

Similarly, "estrogen receptor negative" breast cancer refers to cells that *do not respond* to estrogen. Only about 23 percent of women have "estrogen receptor negative" cancers, therefore circulating estrogen levels in the blood should be of great interest to most women with breast cancer.

All women have estrogen and it varies only by degree. Premenopausal women produce higher levels of estrogen than postmenopausal women. Because estrogen will speed up the growth of hormonally driven cancers the amount of estrogen in the system becomes important. Women with high estrogen levels have faster growing breast cancers than women with lower estrogen levels.

In a study that evaluated the effect of diet and nutrition on cancer, Dr. Lu, Ph.D., Associate Professor, and colleagues, at the University of Texas Medical Branch in Galveston, Texas, investigated the effect of soybean consumption on breast cancer. Previous research had demonstrated that eating soybeans was associated with reduced risk for breast cancer influenced by estrogen. Dr. Lu and her colleagues attempted to explain this finding by looking at the effect of soybean consumption on the body's circulating levels of estrogen.

The research team found that blood levels of measured estrogens were reduced by 30-40 percent in women who consumed soybeans. This led them to conclude that women who consume soybeans reduce their circulating levels of estrogen. "Reducing estrogen reduces breast cell proliferation," said Dr. Lu. "This may help explain why soybean consumption seems to protect against breast cancer."[5]

Besides phytoestrogens, research on soy has isolated several anticancer compounds in the whole soybean that may be beneficial to breast and other cancer patients. Not all of these anticancer compounds have the same mechanisms of action. Since this section is focused on the soy phytoestrogens, the following mechanisms of action may benefit the breast cancer patient regardless of their estrogen level:

- AntiCancer actions of phytoestrogens
- Estrogen-like actions
  Selective Estrogen Receptor – Beta agonism
  Estrogen Antagonism
  MCF-7 cell proliferation
- Modulation of sex steroid metabolism
  Decreased serum estradiol, 16-hydroxyestrogens
  Inhibition of enzymes of estradiol biosynthesis
  Sulfatase/sulfotransferase inhibition
  Enhanced SHBG synthesis
- Anti-proliferative/apoptotic actions
  Inhibition of protein tyrosine kinase
  Antioxidant activity
  Inhibition of DNA topoisomerase
  Induction of tumor cell differentiation,
    G2/M arrest
  Induction of TGF- Beta 1, WAF1/C1P1
  Suppression of COX, C-FOS, heat shock protein
  Inhibition of angiogenesis

Since this chapter deals with "estrogen positive" breast cancer we will focus on the estrogen-like anticancer actions listed above.

---

[5] Lu, Lee, Jane, W., "Soybean. Diet and Breast Cancer Prevention," *Citations from Federal Research in Progress (FRP)*, Univ. Texas Medical Branch, Galveston, TX, FRP 02-12 5M01RR00073-390443 NDN-049-0482-8954-3.

Selective Estrogen Receptor Beta Agonism:

For estrogen or estrogen-like compounds to exert an estrogenic effect they must bind to an estrogen receptor site in cells. The soy phytoestrogens genistein and daidzein are similar to 17 Beta-Estradiol in their structure but they are 100,000 fold weaker in estrogenic activity. Plant estrogens are called phytoestrogens and cause biological effects similar to estrogen. However, because they are very weak estrogens they bind to estrogen receptor sites with less affinity than the hormone estrogen. Although the isoflavones are weak estrogens, people who eat soy foods or products can have blood levels of isoflavones as much as 10,000 times higher than those who do not consume the soy. The higher concentrations of isoflavones in the blood, offsets the weak estrogen-like effects and can have a therapeutic effect at high levels.

There are two estrogen receptor-binding sites that play a role in the effect of estrogen and estrogenic compounds. These receptor sites are known as estrogen-receptor-Alpha and the second is known as estrogen-receptor-Beta. Soybean isoflavones bind with strong affinity, almost as great as estrogen, to the Estrogen-Receptor-Beta site but, with weak affinity to the Estrogen-Receptor-Alpha site. One study showed that binding to the Estrogen-Receptor-Beta site exerts an anticancer effect.[6]

Isoflavones

Weak estrogens, like isoflavones, act not as estrogens but as antiestrogens. This action was considered to be a factor in soy consuming countries for the low breast cancer mortality rates. It was also noted that Japanese breast cancer patients have better survival results than those consuming Western diets.

---

[6] Drs. Lazennec, G., Bresson, D., Lucas, A., Chauveau, C., Vignon, F., "ER Beta Inhibits Proliferation and Invasion of Breast Cancer Cells," *Endocrinology*, 2001: 142:4120-30.

Isoflavones may exert antiestrogenic effects in any of the following ways:

- Competing with estrogen for binding to the estrogen receptor sites;
- Down-regulation of estrogen receptors; thus fewer estrogen receptors are available to which estrogen can bind;
- Increasing serum levels of sex hormone binding globulin (SHBG). SHGB is the protein in serum that carries estrogen. More SHBG means more estrogen in bound in the serum, and less is available to bind to estrogen receptors in cells;
- Altering the metabolism of estrogen in a way that makes estrogen less estrogenic and carcinogenic;
- Decreasing the synthesis of estrogen, thereby decreasing serum estrogen levels;
- Altering the estrogen receptor so it is less able to bind estrogen;
- Inhibiting the post-receptor (after binding) effects of estrogen.

At low concentrations both tamoxifen and the soy isoflavone *genistein* stimulate the growth of estrogen receptor-positive breast cancer cells but, does not stimulate the growth of estrogen receptor-negative breast cancer cells. At high concentrations the soy isoflavone geinstein inhibits the growth of both types of breast cancer cells.[7]

No studies have found that soy or isoflavones actually increase mammary carcinogenesis in rodents who were administered a mammary carcinogen. In addition, as stated on the website talksoy.com, more than twenty human studies have found that a single serving of soy per day does reduce

---

[7] Peterson, G., Barnes, S., "Genistein Inhibition of The Growth of Human Breast Cancer Cells Independence from Estrogen Receptors. The Multi-Drug Resistance Gene," *Biochem Biophys Res Commun* 1991; 179:661-7 and Peterson, G., Barnes, S., "Genistein Inhibits Both Estrogen and Growth Factor-Stimulated Proliferation of Human Breast Cancer Cells." *Cell Growth Differ*, 1996;7:1345-51.

cancer risk. This helps to assure users that soy is not harmful to estrogen receptor-positive breast cancer patients. In addition, two studies found that soy acted either additively or synergistically with the breast cancer drug tamoxifen to inhibit the development of mammary tumors in rats. One of those studies found that by combining soy and tamoxifen, the growth of existing mammary tumors in rats was inhibited, whereas tamoxifen by itself was ineffective.[8] The other study from the University of Illinois showed the effectiveness of tamoxifen by itself was 26 percent, soy protein isolate by itself was 36 percent and the two together were 62 percent. The hypothesis for the two working better together than either one individually is attributed to the fact that the soy has a stronger affinity for the beta receptor sites than the tamoxifen. Ttamosifen on the other hand has a stronger affinity to the alpha receptor site. Therefore, the two together have more effective blocking on both the alpha and beta receptor sites than either one individually.[9]

The missing link – estrogen metabolism!

Some estrogen metabolites damage DNA and are clearly carcinogenic. Therefore, it is important to focus on not only the levels of circulating estrogens in the body, but the metabolites of estrogens present, their quantities and the ratios existing between these estrogen metabolites. Recent studies have focused on a number of estrogen metabolites. Two of these, 4-hydroxestrone, and 16-a-hydroxyestrone, are genetosic, mutagenic and procarcinogenic. On the other hand 2-methoxyestrone has very weak estrogenic properties; 2-methoxy-estradiol, which is normally present in the body in

---

[8]Gotoh T. Yamada K, Ito A. Yin H, Kataoka T, Dohi K., "Chemoprevention of N-nitroso-N-metylurea-induced rat mammary cancer by miso and tamoxifen, alone and in combination," *Jpn J Cancer Res*, 1998; 89:487-95.
[9] Constantinou AI, Xu H, Lucas LM, Lanjvit D. Soy Enhances Tamoxifen's cancer chemopreventitive effects in female rats, Fourth International Symposium on the Role of Soy in Preventing and Treating Chronic disease, November 4-7, 2001, San Diego, CA.

trace elements has significant anticancer properties. Based on the different effects of these estrogen metabolites, Bradlow and colleagues developed the urinary estrogen metabolite ratio test, to evaluate a patient's balance of "good" (2-hydroxy) and "bad" (16-hydroxy) (ref #1) estrogens.[10] Studies in premenopausal caucasian women showed that a higher 2/16 metabolite ratio was associated with a decreased risk of estrogen-related cancers.[11] In one major Italian study higher 2/16 estrogen metabolite ratios were associated with a reduction in breast cancer in premenopausal women, but higher ratios in postmenopausal women were associated with an increased risk of breast cancer.[12]

Studies show that the whole soy not only reduces the levels of circulating estrogens, but in addition improves the 2/16 estrogen metabolite ratios. In one study the 16 hydroxy estrogens were reduced 81 percent by the soy. Major testing laboratories in many countries now offer estrogen metabolism testing. It was concluded that a ratio of two or more times the 2-hydroxy estrogens vs. the 16 hydroxy estrogens places women in a low risk category for breast cancers. It should also be noted that in addition to the estrogen metabolites cited above there are other metabolites that exist. Of those, Equol is a fermentation product of the soy phytoestrogen daidzein. Equol production is associated with a reduced risk of breast cancer and other estrogen-mediated cancers, improved bone mineral density, and may also have cardio-

---

[10] Meilahn EN, De Stavola B, Allen DS, Fentiman I, Bradlow HL, Sepkovic DW, Kuller LH. Do urinary oestrogen metabolites predict breast cancer? Guernsey III cohort follow-up. Br J Cancer. 1998Nov; 78(9):1250-5.

[11] Loard RS, Bongiovanni B, Bralley JA, Estrogen metabolism and the diet-cancer connection; rationale for assessing the ratio of urinary hydroxylated estrogen metabolites. Alter Med Rev. 2002 Apr; 7(2):112-29/ Review.

[12] I Muti P, Bradlow HL, Micheli A, Krogh V, Freudenheim JL, Schunemann HJ, Stanulla M, Yang J, Sepkovic DW, Trevisan M, Berrino F. Estrogen metabolism and risk of breast cancer; a prospective study of the 2:16 alpha-hydroxyestrone ratio in premenopausal and postmenopausal women. Epidemiology. 2000 Nov; 11(6):635-40.

vascular benefits as well. Many researchers are now changing their focus from genistein and daidzein to Equol as a key "active" component in soy's effectiveness. Since Equol is a gut fermentation product only those with the required intestinal microflora are equol producers. Infants have been shown lacking in the ability to produce Equol but acquire the ability sometime after four months of age – presumably by acquiring the appropriate gut flora during the first year of their life. Antibiotics have been shown to destroy the gut flora required for Equol production. It can take four to six months to reestablish the gut flora in order to restore Equol production.

Refuting negative study on soy promoting cancer

There are other in vitro (test tube) and rat studies that are inconclusive as to the beneficial or harmful effects of soy isoflavones. However, an animal study that has caused a lot of concern and confusion on the issue of soy and breast health, concluded that soy promoted the growth of "estrogen receptor positive" breast cancers. The researchers at the University of Illinois, conducted the study by the following:

- Used immune deficient mice who had their ovaries removed, which stopped their production of estrogen;
- Implanted them with actual "estrogen receptor positive" breast cancer cells (rather than being exposed to a carcinogen);
- Gave them genistein, (tumor growth is stimulated in comparison to mice not given genistein). Soy protein isolate also has this effect, although both the effects of genistein and isolate are much less than estrogen.

It is unfortunate, but this flawed study has prevented the majority of researchers and doctors from recommending the use of soy products to women with estrogen receptor positive breast cancers. When asked what was wrong with the study, critics presented the following reasons for not considering its significance:

>The design of the study is taken from the model used for determining the anticancer effect of chemotherapy drugs. The rats in this animal study are immune-system deficient in order to eliminate tumor shrinkage that is a result of any immune stimulation properties of the item being tested. This is a fine animal model for chemotherapy drugs that normally destroy the immune system, but it is a definite handicap to any product that does not destroy immune function. For example, Haelan's fermented soy beverage increases nonspecific immunity 700 percent, which produces tumor shrinkage, fewer animal deaths, and longer animal life spans.

Note: The animal model described favors toxic chemotherapy drugs. When you destroy the immune system's capability, the toxic chemotherapy drugs will always get greater tumor shrinkage than any nontoxic therapy, which relies to a great extent on immune-stimulating properties for tumor shrinkage and promoting longer life spans.

>Other researchers have found that when the ovaries of the rats are not surgically removed genistein has the opposite effect. It actually markedly inhibits mammary tumor development in rodents implanted with estrogen receptor-positive breast cancer cells. In other words, if a continuing supply of estrogen were present in a control group the tumors in the soy-supplemented rats would have been much smaller than those in the non-soy supplemented group. This is a significant issue when we take into consideration that the study by Dr. Lu, and colleagues at the University of Texas Medical Branch in Galveston, Texas showed that circulating estrogen levels are 30-40 percent lower in women who consumed soybeans. Therefore, a realistic study would have included a comparison using soy-supplemented rats with a continued estrogen supply compared to a control group of rats with a continued estrogen supply but with no soy supplementation.[13]

---

[13] Shao, A.M., Wu, J., Shen, Z.Z., Barsky, S.H., "Genistein Exerts Multiple Suppressive Effects on Human Breast Carcinoma Cells," *Cancer Res* 1998L 58:4851-7; and Zhou, J.R., "Prevention of Orthotropic Growth of Estrogen-Dependent Human Breast Tumor In Mice by Dietary Soy Phy-

Progestins and HRT

There is growing support that synthetic progesterone and progestins are the culprits in increasing breast cancer risks in women who have been taking hormone replacement therapy (HRT). Women who have an intact uterus have been taking synthetic estrogen plus another hormone produced by the ovaries, progesterone in an unnatural form manufactured as progestins (medroxy progesterone). This is because estrogen by itself increases the risk of endometrial cancer, whereas estrogen plus progesterone does not.

Hormone replacement therapy (HRT) containing estrogens and progestins has been associated with a 2-3 fold increased breast cancer risk over a women's lifetime, whereas estrogen by itself is only weakly associated with an increased risk of cancer. Biological data suggests that progestins used in HRT prescriptions have a harmful effect on breast tissue, whereas soy improves breast tissue health, because soy isoflavones have no progesterone activity.

The use of natural progesterone cannot be equated with the risks of progestin used in HRT. Research shows that women with low progesterone have up to 500 percent more risk of early breast cancer and may warrant supplementation.[14] Transdermal applications of natural progesterone has shown to balance hormone insufficiencies as well as guard against bone loss, normalize blood pressure, decrease heart disease, and resist cancer.[15]

No risk soy

Mark Messina, Ph.D., M.S., stated "the evidence overall suggests that soy will not have detrimental effects when consumed by breast cancer patients. Consequently, breast cancer patients for whom soy products are an important part of the diet need not stop using them. Although the evidence is not sufficient at this time to recommend that

---

tochemicals," *222nd American Chemical Society Meeting.* Chicago, Illinois 2001: Abstract 121.

[14] Am Jnl Epidemiology, 1981, vol 114.

[15] Mason, Roger, *No More Horse Estrogen*, Safe Goods, 2001.

breast cancer patients begin to consume soyfoods specifically for the purposes of enhancing survival, much evidence suggests soy exerts other benefits that warrant its use."[16]

On the subject of "estrogen receptor positive" breast cancer, and others, it is important to point out that when tumor studies are done on isoflavones by themselves, there is less tumor shrinkage compared to studies on whole soybean where the isoflavone components are removed. The soy matrix contains many anticancer compounds and their synergistic effects are superior to the soy isoflavones, or any other soy isolates by themselves. Therefore, the results of in vitro (test tube) and the animal studies cited that use isoflavones by themselves are not indicative of the results that might be achieved if a concentrated whole soy fermented beverage had been used in the study.[17]

---

[16] Messina, M., Barnes, S., "The Role of Soy Products in Reducing Risk of Cancer," *J Natl Cancer Inst*, 1991, 83, 541-546.
[17] Ibid.

4

SOY—*its benefit and . . .*
The fermented or unfermented controversy?

Soy has gained a foothold in the American diet. From May 2000 to May 2001 natural products stores sold over $14 million worth of soy supplements and almost $219 million in soy meal replacements and supplement powders, according to SPINS, a market research firm that provides information to the health and wellness industry. The World Health Organization reported in the year 2000[18] that the Japanese, with their extensive consumption of *cultured* soy products, such as miso, natto, tempeh, and accompanying foods such as ginger, ocean herbs, and green tea have the longest healthy life expectancy of any people on earth. Soybeans are one of nature's highest sources of nutrients, especially protein. They are rich in anticarcinogenic compounds, particularly isoflavones like genistein and daidzein. Reports conclude that as little as one serving of soy foods per day can protect people against cancers of the lung, colon, rectum, stomach, prostate, and breast.

There are two schools of thinking about soy in our diets. There is support based on soy products contributing to a low incidence of some cancers, based on health statistics, particularly from the Orient. Many have used this as a marketing enticement for consumers to use soy as a high-integrity protein, substituting it for the meat and dairy in their diets. Foods traditionally used in the Orient are derived from fermented soy products. Soy foods we see produced commercially are normally derived from nonfermented soy. There is a difference.

Traditional nonfermented soy foods include fresh green soybeans, whole dry soybeans, soy nuts, whole fat soy flour,

[18]"WHO issues New Healthy Life Expectancy Rankings," *Press release,* World Health Organization 2000, June 2000, Washington D.C. and Geneva, Switzerland.

soymilk, and tofu. Fermented soy foods include tempeh, miso, soy sauces, natto, fermented tofu, and fermented soymilk. The traditional fermentation process serves several functions, including the enrichment of food substrates biologically with protein, essential amino acids, essential fatty acids, vitamins, polyamines, carbohydrates, and numerous anti-oxidants and phytosterols.[19] In Asia, fermented soy foods are considered to have more health promoting benefits than nonfermented products consumed in the West.[20] The fermentation process, for example, with lactobacilli, increases the quantity, availability, digestibility, and assimilation of nutrients in the body.[21] Studies done on the effect of miso on cancer, for example, concluded that it was the culturing process itself that led to a lowered number of cancers per animal and reduced tumour growth rates compared to the control group. It was determined that the effect was caused by the cultured soy medium itself being rich in the isoflavone aglycones, genistein, and daizein which are believed to be cancer chemopreventives.[22]

Soy is a difficult food to digest and therefore many of its benefits never reach their destination. Only 3-5 percent can be broken down, making it difficult for the liver and kidneys, which must flush the excess from the body. The coating on the soybean contains trypsin inhibitors that prevent the normal digestive processes from breaking it down. In test studies with animals, diets high in trypsin inhibitors cause enlargement and pathological conditions of the pancreas, including cancer. When the soybean is sprouted or fermented, the trypsin inhibitors become insignificant.

---

[19] Haard N, Odunfa SA, Lee C etal., *Fermented cereals: A global perspective*. Food and Agricultural Organisation of the United Nations Rome, 1999.
[20] Ibid.
[21] Gorbach SL., Lactic acid bacteria and human health. *Annals of Internal Medicine*, 1990; 22 (1): 37-41.
[22] Baggott, J.E., Ha, T.,Vaughn, W.H., Et. al., "Effect of miso and NaCl on DMBA-induced rat mammary tumors, *Nutr Cancer*, 1990; 14(2): 103-9.

Tofu has reduced levels of the inhibitors, as most of them precipitate out of the bean curd into the soaking liquid. Therefore, tofu may be easier to digest than soymilk, although the trypsin inhibitors are reduced, but not totally eliminated. In many cases, supplemental enzymes, specifically protease,[23] may be needed to digest unfermented soy. When a manufacturer ferments soy, it is broken down to an amino acid stage that goes beyond what the body's digestion can do alone. Traditionally, Asians have sprouted or fermented their soybeans prior to eating them. This process breaks down the food components into smaller particles, knocks out the growth-stunting components, and deactivates the chemotrypsin-blocking effects of the protease inhibitors in soy. Therefore, the food becomes digestible and beneficial allowing the release of its numerous nutrients. Foods such as tempe and miso, sprouted soy powders and fermented soy liquid concentrates, are easily digested.

The cultured bean contains isoflavones—notably, genistein and daidzein complexes—as well as vitamin E and quercetin. The fermentation process is thought to convert the *precursors of* genistein and daidzein in the complexes to the *actively* anticancer forms of genistein and daidzein. Studies on cultured soybeans have shown that the phytonutrients and cofactors may neutralize the damaging effects of many carcinogenic compounds. A Japanese study found that the level of genistein in the fermented soybean products was higher than in unfermented soybeans and soybean products such as soymilk and tofu.[24]

Tofu and soy products contain a high concentration of isoflavones but to obtain therapeutic levels you would have to eat more than half a pound of tofu to reach the recommended health maintenance levels of 50-80mg daily of

---

[23] Plant-based enzymes that are organically grown are preferable.

[24] Grun, I.U., Adhikari, K., Li, C., et al., "Changes in the profile of genistein, daidzein and their conjugates during thermal processing of tofu," *J Agric Food Chem,* June 2001; 49(6):2839-43.

the beneficial isoflavone genistein.[25] Fermented and sprouted soy supplementation because of their digestibility is a superior method of providing the body with the micronutrients of soy.

Many of the constituents in soy have beneficial effects in fighting cancer. The National Cancer Institute studied the anticancer compounds in fruit and vegetables and found five super star anticancer compounds, all of which are found abundantly in soybeans.[26] The five are isoflavones, protease inhibitors, saponins, phytosterols and phytic acid compounds. One of these anticancer compounds, isoflavones has nine metabolites (genestein, acetyl genestin, glycitein, malonyl glycitin, malonyl daidzin, genistin, glycitin, and daidzin.) Genestine alone has had more than 600 clinical studies dealing with various forms of cancer.

Isoflavones have the ability to shut down the blood supply that feeds the cancer cells. Therefore, the tumors shrink and die because they have no food supply (a process known as anti-angiogenesis). Isoflavones also have the ability to induce the normal form of cell death that leads to the disintegration of cells into membrane-bound particles (apoptosis). These particles are then removed from the body by white blood cells, called macrophage, which engulf and break down the cell particles for removal from the body. Apoptosis is a non-toxic method of restoring the death of cancer cells that have lost the ability to die when they have offspring (resulting in tumor growth). Isoflavones also have the ability to reverse some nonnormal cells to a normal condition by repairing the cell's DNA decreasing levels of oxidative DNA damage in humans.[27]

Isoflavones by themselves, although impressive in their tumor- shrinkage capability, do not shrink tumors better than the whole soy with the isoflavones removed. Therefore,

---

[25] Holt, Steven, M.D., *Soya for Health: The Definitive Medical Guide,* 1996, Ann Liebert, Inc.

[26] Journal of the National Cancer Institute, April 17, 1991, vol. 83 No. 8.

[27] Marnett, L. Oxyradicals and DNA Damage, *Carcinogenesis,* 2000; 21:361-370.

the tumor-shrinking capability of the other anticancer compounds in soy, when used together, are greater than the ability of the isoflavones to shrink tumors when used alone.

Soy's Bowman-Birk protease inhibitor (BBI) has been proven to prevent the activation of genes that can cause cancer. Isoflavones known as "phytoestrogens," resembling estradiol, an estrogen found in the body whose excess has been linked certain types of cancer, also have antiestrogen properties. Soy isoflavones have the ability to stimulate differentiation, causing cancerous cells to change back into healthy, noncancerous cells, and the isoflavones also inhibit cancer cell growth.[28] Isoflavones mimic estrogen in the body, but they are significantly less potent in comparison to natural estrogens. These isoflavones, or phytoestrogens, are successful at competing for the hormone receptor sites and as a result, cellular estrogen levels decrease. Please note that these are only more successful for estrogen beta-receptor sites, not alpha sites. Since many cancers are related to excess estrogen concentrations, this helps prevent estrogen buildup.

The cultured bean contains naturally occurring isoflavones—notably, gonistein and daidzein complexes—as well as vitamin E and quercetin. The fermentation process is thought to convert the isoflavone *precursors* genistein and daidzein to their *active* anticancer isoflavone forms genistein and daidzein. Studies on cultured soybeans have shown that the beneficial effects of the phytonutrients and cofactors may neutralize the damaging effects of many carcinogenic compounds. A Japanese study found that the level of genistein in the fermented soybean products was higher than in soybeans and soybean products such as nonfermented soymilk and tofu.[29]

---

[28] Divi, R.L., Chang, H.C., "Anti-thyroid isoflavones from soybean: isolation, characterization, and mechanisms of action, *Biochem Pharmacol*, 1997, Nov. 15; 54 (10):1087-96.

[29] Grun, I.U., Adhikari, K., Li, C., et al., "Changes in the profile of genistein, daidzein and their conjugates during thermal processing of tofu," *J Agric Food Chem*, June 2001; 49(6):2839-43.

Sprouted or fermented soy is more effective in the healing process, if it is mineral-rich and harvested at its peak phytochemical content. There are over 10,000 known varieties of soybeans. Their nutritional value has been documented to vary up to 50 percent, and that variation is thought to be based on several factors. Minerals carry nutrients; therefore, if the soil where they are grown is compromised or depleted of important minerals, the soy crop will be nutrient-deficient. Another factor is the harvesting period. Harvesting the soy crop at specific times will also cause the nutrient quality to vary. The beans must be harvested at the peak of phytochemical production, which has been determined from harvesting research. Therefore, sprouted or fermented soy, if it is grown on mineral rich soil and harvested at its peak phytochemical content, has the nutrient "blueprint" to contribute to optimum healing results.

Eating cultured soybean products will deliver a more concentrated form of the beneficial compounds than processed soy foods. Supplements made from soy sprouts must be made with a low-temperature drying process, as heat denatures the vital enzymes and nutrients of the soy. Fermented soy concentrates, supplements, and powders will deliver higher levels of active, beneficial nutrients, because soy's beneficial properties become available to the body, once the bean has been digested. The fermented liquid-soy concentrate used by the cancer patients in the next chapter, not only contains all the benefits listed below, but has a delivery system that gets anticancer agents into the cancer cell.

Summary

Healing properties of this potent bean:
▸ Prevents activation of cancer-causing genes
▸ Inhibits tumor growth
▸ Prevents heart and cardiovascular disease
▸ Increases the number and activity of killer cells

▸ Neutralizes free-radicals
▸ Lowers cholesterol
▸ Good source of lecithin and Omega-3 fatty acids
▸ Excessive estrogen-blocker
▸ Reduces circulating estrogen levels and improves estrogen metabolism ratio of "good" estrogens vs. "bad" estrogens.
▸ Reduces blood flow to the tumor
▸ Guards against bone loss and osteoporosis
▸ Effective anti-inflammatory
▸ Anti-viral components

These healing properties are due to the many soybean constituents, but principally to those noted in the following discussion. It must again be emphasized that to be most effective the soybean must be in a digestible state—**fermented or sprouted**.

• Protease inhibitors: a phytochemical that prevents conversion of normal cells to the malignant state, even at very late stages in carcinogenesis (not related to the protease enzyme). Protease inhibitors have no effect on canccrous cells.[30] Protease inhibitors can be found in potatoes, eggs, and cereals, although, when these foods are cooked, the phytochemicals are destroyed. Soybeans have an abundance of protease inhibitors, which seem to survive even after heating.

• Phytates: a phytochemical that inhibits tumor growth in a wide range of cancers, as well as preventing heart and cardivascular disease. They enhance overall immunity by increasing the number and activity of cells, whose job is to kill foreign or noncomplying cells. They also act as antioxidants to bind with iron in the intestines, preventing the production of free radicals. In addition, they slow down the "doubling rate" of cancer cell growth (a process called mitosis).

---

[30] Kennedy, A. R., *Carcinogenesis*, 6:1441-1445, 1985.

• Phytosterols: sterols obtained from plants that help control cholesterol, and inhibit the development of colon and skin tumors.

• Saponins: antioxidants that neutralize free radicals and prevent cellular mutations that could lead to cancer. In one study, when mixed with H.I.V., they stopped the virus from replicating. Saponins can also lower cholesterol.

• Phenolic Acids: antioxidant that prevents cellular DNA from being attacked by carcinogens.

• Lecithin: a phosphorus-rich fat that is essential for transforming other fats in the body so they can be absorbed. It also is used to lower cholesterol, reduce the incidence of tumors, and to support the brain, central nervous, and immune systems.

• Omega-3 fatty acids: unsaturated fats that are needed by the body to protect against heart disease (reduces plaque), support the liver, nourish the immune system by combining with other nutrients to increase T cell life, and have anti-inflammatory properties.

• Isoflavones (phytoestrogens): plant estrogens that have known anticancer effects on all cancers, but particularly in hormone-related cancers, such as breast, ovarian, and prostate cancer, when caused by high estrogen levels. They are similar in structure to the female hormone estrogen, but are only $1/1000^{th}$ as potent, and are known as weak estrogens. They have the ability to block the uptake of estrogen by estrogen-sensitive tissues, in cases where excessive estrogen levels are present, caused by the consumption of hormone-fed livestock or certain pesticide-treated fruits and vegetables. As mentioned before, two specific isoflavones and their metabolites, have extremely beneficial anticancer properties. These are genistein and daidzein.

Genistein:
1. blocks the uptake of estrogen; (however, not found in breast tissue —daidzein is found there);

2. prevents cancer cell growth by inhibiting the activity of enzymes, which further the growth of cancer;
3. causes cancer cells to convert to normal cells. A normal cell becomes cancerous when it becomes more primitive. Genistein reverses this process;
4. inhibits angiogenesis (blood supply that nourishes the cancer cells), causing the tumor to starve to death;
5. acts as a powerful antioxidant;
6. prevents DNA damage in healthy cells;

Daidzein:
1. guards against bone loss and the development of osteoporosis;
2. powerful antioxidant;
3. anticancer agent;
4. replacement for estrogen supplementation.
5. is found in breast tissue;
6. a pre-cursor to the phytoestrogen "Equol."

Healthy-heart benefits of fermented soy

There are nine primary benefits of soy products for a healthy heart. Other benefits are possible but the extent of the benefits depends on the processing of the soy product because all soy products are not equal in composition nor are they processed alike. Therefore, other cardiovascular benefits vary by both degree and extent of the benefits.

- Ace Inhibitory Effect of Soy Nutrients
  Soy contains phytonutrients that strongly inhibit the angiotensin-converting enzyme ("ACE") and therefore promotes heart health. ACE inhibitors represent a significant class of pharmaceuticals, but researchers from the Tokyo University of Agriculture in 1995 confirmed that fermented soy did an effective job at the same task.

- Restores of elasticity of arteries
  Soy has been shown to restore the elasticity of the arteries. This promotes lower blood pressure and improved long-term heart health.

- Prevents the profileration and migration of foam cells
  Clinical trials have shown a reduction (approx. 66%) in the profileration and migration of "foam" cells in the arteries. Foam cells form blockages in the arteries and contribute to heart attacks. A reduction in their formation and migration is consistent with heart health.

- Cholesterol lowering capability
  The fermentation of a food has been shown to cause an increase in human gut "friendly" bacterial content. Once they are living in the large intestine these rich

in soy bacteria are believed to ferment indigestible carbohydrates. This fermentation causes increased production of short-chain fatty acids, which decease circulatory cholesterol concentrations either by inhibiting hepatic cholesterol syntheses or by redistributing cholesterol from plasma to the liver. (NOTE: Nagata C, Takatsuka N, Kurisu Y, Shimizu H. Decreased serum total cholesterol concentration is associated with high intake of soy products in Japanese men and women.[31] In addition, increased bacterial activity in the large intestine results in enhanced bile acid deconjugation which are not well absorbed by the gut mucosa and are excreted along with the cholesterol. These actions combined are proposed as contributing mechanisms of fermented soy to decrease circulating cholesterol concentrations.

- Improvement in heart function
  The left power pump output of the heart was increased in studies with humans who took part in an anti-aging study[32] using Haelan's fermented soy beverage. In addition, it was shown that blood oxygen content was increased as well as the antioxidant index of the circulating blood. These are significant contributing factors promoting heart health.

- Improvement in Lung Function
  Clinical trials with humans using Haelan's fermented soy products were shown to have improved volumetric lung functioning.[33] In addition, higher oxygen content in the circulating blood was experienced. These factors are consistent with improvement in heart health.

---

[31] J Nutr. 1998; 128:209-213
[32] U.S. RESEARCH REPORT NO. 101
[33] U.S. RESEARCH REPORT NO 101

- Vasodilation
  Clinical trials have shown vasodilation properties of fermented soy.[34] The micro-circulation half time rate of circulating blood in humans was reduced, which is consistent with heart health.

- Anti-oxidant Protection
  Cardiologist at a research hosital in Kyoto, Japan determined that fermentation changed the biological activity of flavonoids. "A significant antioxidant activity has been found in fermented soy suggesting that the soy flavonoids can be absorbed from the intestine more efficiently than unfermented soy. The fermenting process enhances cardiovascular antioxidant availability."[35]

- Blood pressure Effects
  In clinical studies fermented soy has been shown to increase kidney blood flow and filtering which is consistent with the maintenance of lower blood pressure and improved cardiovascular health.

[34] Shimokado,K., Yokota, T., Umezawa,K., Sasaguri, T., Ogata, J., 1994, Arterioscler. Thromb. 14, ppp.973-981.
[35] Tikkanen, M.J., Wahala,K., Ojala, S., Vibrna, V. Aldercreutz, H., 1995, In 68th Scientific Sessions of the American Heart Assn. Abstract.

6

Personal Success Stories

The testimonials in this chapter lay claim to the value of a specific nutrient that we have discovered can make the difference between surviving cancer or being a casualty. The healing power of the soyfoods varies widely, with cultured varieties providing more nutrient absorption. The soy beverage used by the following survivors is made from a patented fermentation procedure. This process hydrolyzes many of the soybean proteins into amino acids and compounds that are rich in nitrogen, polysaccharides, and fermentation metabolites of the naturally occurring isoflavones, protease inhibitors, saponins, phytosterols, and inositol hexaphosphate compounds in soybeans.

The soy beverage is a concentrated nutritional supplement that is rich in soybean proteins, selenium, zinc, beta-carotene (vitamin A), riboflavin (B-1), thiamine (B-2), cyanocobalamin (B-12), vitamin C as ascorbate, cholecalciferol (D-3), alphatocopherol (E), and phylloquinone (K-1). It also contains additional micronutrients such as daidzein, genistein, protease inhibitors, saponins, phytosterols and inositol hexaphosphate, essential fatty acids (linolenic and linoleic acids), polysaccharide peptide, and twenty of the twenty-two amino acids including ornithine.[36] Of these naturally occurring nutritional items, more than twenty of them are known individually for their ability to enhance the nutritional profiles of individuals with cancers.[37] The survival rate of cancer patients using a soy phytochemical beverage can give all of us hope that this disease does not have to have a death sentence attached to it. The following stories directly

---

[36] "Quality analysis report on Haelan 951, 2001," *Central Analytical Laboratories, Inc.*, 101 Woodland Hwy, Belle Chasse, LA, 70037.
[37] Nair, Vijaya, M.D., M.S., and Vic Hernandez, M.P.H., "A Novel Fermented Soya Beverage and Safe Nutritive Adjunct in Prostate Cancer Therapies: Is There a Possible Chemopreventive Role?, *Townsend Letter for Doctors & Patients,* July, 2002.

from the cancer survivors depict how traditional treatments as well as the soy beverage can have miraculous results.

Breast and ovarian cancer

Women have a strong impetus to find a cure for breast cancer, but to avoid becoming a statistic, they should also look at the potential causes. Greater lifelong exposure to estrogen is thought to increase breast cancer risk. Hidden cancer cells can remain dormant in a woman's body for years, just waiting for estrogen to start stimulating them. Chemical estrogenic substances such as found in chemicals and pesticides may trigger activation. Poor diets, mineral deficiencies, stress, and negative emotions can put the body's defenses (the immune system) in a weakened state and vulnerable to cancer growth. Earlier age at menses and later age at menopause are considered high risk factors.[38] This is why doctors recommend estrogen-sensitive breast cancer patients not use HRT (hormone replacement therapy.) Because soybean phytoestrogens act as a weak estrogen, there has been concern as to its safety as a "hormone replacement."

Although isoflavones (considered phytoestrogens) found in soy bind to estrogen receptors, they do so at a weakened level and seem to be selective. They exert estrogen-like effects on the bone and coronary vessels, but not on endometrial tissue. This contrasts with estrogen, which has an estrogenic effect on all tissues and appears to increase the risk of breast and endometrial cancer.[39] The tissue selective effects of isoflavones have led many experts to classify them as natural selective estrogen receptor modulators, for which

---

[38] Morabia, A., Costanza, M.C., "International variability in ages at menarche, first livebirth and menopause, World Health Organization Collaborative Study of Neoplasia and Steroid Contraceptives," [published erratum appears in Am J Epidemiol, Sept 1999; 150 (5):546], *Am J Epidemiol*, 1998, 148:1195-205.

[39] Persson, I., "Estrogens in the causation of breast, endometrial and ovarian cancers – evidence and hypotheses from epidemiological findings," *J Steroid Biochem Mol Biol*, 2000; 74:357-64.

pharmaceutical companies are currently modeling drugs after. The breast cancer drug tamoxifen is one of these because it exerts estrogenic effects on the bones and blood vessels, but antiestrogenic effects on the breast. The drug's value is diminished when you consider the many side effects, such as endometrial cancer.

Isoflavones may exert antiestrogenic effects through competitive binding. This means it must first bind to estrogen receptors to affect cells. Isoflavones do bind to these receptors, but their effect is much weaker than estrogen and since they compete with estrogen for binding to the estrogen receptors, if sufficient amounts of isoflavones are consumed, they will occupy the receptor sites instead of the estrogen. This indicates they may actually be antiestrogenic. In studies examining soy isoflavones effect on breast cancer in animals, researchers found that the addition of soy to the diet does not necessarily significantly inhibit tumor incidence. They did find that it inhibited tumor multiplicity by 15-50 percent regarding phytic acid input on both frequency and size of tumor.[40] Other studies found that Chinese women, who consumed soy as young girls, are about 50 percent less likely to develop breast cancer later in life.[41]

Advanced breast cancer
Nina P., a senior, is a breast cancer survivor. In 1996 she was diagnosed with advanced breast cancer, which had metastasized to her clavicle, hips, and spine. The doctors offered surgery, which she promptly refused. She decided not to undergo radiation or chemotherapy, choosing instead an alternative route. She made lifestyle changes, and started drinking a soy concentrate daily. Three months later, her doctor was shocked to find no signs of cancer. Three years later, her

[40] Goyoh, T., Yamada K., Yin, H., Ito, A., Kataoka, T., Dohi, K., "Chemoprevention of N-nitroso-N-methylurea-induced rat mammary carcinogenesis by soy foods or biochanin, A. Jpn," *J Cancer Res,* 1998; 89: 137-42.
[41] Shu, X.O, Jin, F., Qu, D., et al. "Adolescent soy food intake and other dietary habits," *Proc Am Assoc Cancer Res,* 2000; 41:94 (abstract 602).

mammograms showed the cancer was still in remission. Scar tissue is the only evidence of a tumor, revealed in her Xrays. Her son reports that she has lost excess weight, is more physically active, and her overall constitution has improved. The son also reported that his father, who has suffered from severe Parkinson's disease for a number of years, also began the soy concentrate regimen, and has a 90 percent reduction in his tremors.

Terminal breast cancer
Vickie Fanelli was diagnosed with metastasized breast cancer that had spread to her bones and lining of her lung. A mastectomy was performed and chemotherapy administered. She received three protocols of high dose chemotherapy. During the treatment with chemotherapy the breast cancer grew. Her oncologist said that this was the fastest growing cancer he had ever treated. Her 24 year-old daughter was told the condition was terminal, and was advised to move her mother to a hospice. Instead, she began giving her mother a soybean phytochemical concentrate. Considered to be terminal, Vicki drank the fermented soy beverage as a sole therapy and her tumor shrank in size approximately 75 percent. She used the beverage for eleven months and by July of 2000, she was alive and mobile without any restrictions. Her doctor confirmed her Xrays are normal. She credits the soy concentrate with saving her life, and now encourages other cancer patients to try it.

The National Cancer Institute has accepted the following cases as "sole therapy cured" cases using Haelan's fermented soy beverage.

Estrogen receptor positive breast cancer
Jan H. had been diagnosed with estrogen receptor positive breast cancer. She had metastasis to the lungs, bronchial area, lymph system, bones, and soft tissue. A lump the size of a baseball was under her ribs. Jan had one unsuccessful round of chemotherapy with very little tumor shrinkage and

was told that she was terminal having three months to live and would require chemotherapy for the rest of her short life because the chemotherapy would not get rid of her cancer. Jan decided it was in her best interest not to take any more chemotherapy and drank one bottle per day of Haelan's 951 fermented soy beverage for ten months and then followed that with one half bottle per day for two months. Jan felt great and decided to go get checked and did both a CAT scan and a PET scan and was told she was cancer free on all tests.

Cancer free without surgery

Patty was 64 when she was diagnosed with ductile carcinoma (a 15 cm x 15 cm tumor) that the doctors estimated had been growing in her breast for eight years. Patty had been under extreme stress during this period of time and believes that was a trigger for her cancer's growth. The physician recommended a total mastectomy or a lumpectomy with removal of the lymph nodes under her arm followed by aggressive radiation. Patty agreed to the lumpectomy but refused to let her lymph nodes be removed. She was appalled when other surgeons tried to bully her into having the lymph glands removed. They tried their best to scare her into surgery, but she refused to have either the lumpectomy or the lymph node removal.

Patty was introduced to the soy beverage at a medical symposium attended by her holistic physician husband. In November she began drinking a bottle per day. In addition she eliminated sugar and alcohol, ate primarily raw, organic foods and put an air purifier in her home. Six weeks later she had a mammogram which revealed a significant decrease in tumor size. Her radiologist was amazed. A third mammogram revealed a 50 percent reduction in the vessel supplying nutrients to the minute tumor. She had four more mammograms, and each time the tumor was measured, it had decreased in size. Two years later her mammogram showed only a shadow where the dead tumor once was. Her doctor confirmed that there were no other nodes or other signs of cancer in the breast tissue. All of her organs had been scanned by ultrasound and there was no evidence of metastases. Her radiologist said that in his 32 years, he had never seen this kind of improvement. He was so convinced that he put his wife on the soy beverage to treat her colon and liver cancer.

Prostate cancer

Prostate cancer is the most common type of nonskin cancer found in most men. The American Cancer Society estimated than in the year 2002, there would be 180,000 new cases of prostate cancer in the United States with a projection for mortality of 31,900 men. Prostate cancer may develop as a result of both inherited and environmental factors and well as being a result of race-ethnicity heritage. A number of epidemiological studies have shown that Western type of diets may be a strong environmental risk factor as well.[42] Prostate cancer mortality is very low in Asian countries where soy foods are consumed.[43]

Early detection and treatment is essential to survival. Whether a tumor will grow slowly with no health consequences to the patient, or will grow quickly and become life threatening is difficult to predict. There are also no definitive clinical studies that compare the relative benefits of treating early stage patients with radiation therapy, radical prostatectomy (surgical removal of the entire prostate gland along with nearby tissues), or watchful waiting.[44] Alternative treatments and preventive measures are emerging with more men discovering their successes. The use of a fermented soy

---

[42] Stephens, F.O., "Phytoestrogens and prostate cancer: possible preventive role," *Medical J Aust*, 1997, 167:138-140.

[43] Rose, D.P., Boyar, A.P., Wynder, E.L., "International comparison of mortality rates for the cancer of the breast, ovary, prostate and colon, and per capita food consumption," *Cancer*, 1986: 58: 2363-2371.

[44] Nair, Vijaya, M.D., M.S., and Vic Hernandez, M.P.H., "A Novel Fermented Soya Beverage and Safe Nutritive Adjunct in Prostate Cancer Therapies: Is There a Possible Chemopreventive Role? *Townsend Letter for Doctors & Patients,* July, 2002.

beverage as a chemopreventive agent has both laboratory and clinical relevance. Genistein has antitumor activity in prostate cancer with an effect on a tumor-bearing protein known as epidermal growth factor. The addition of genistein to mammalian cells had down regulated the expression of this receptor and can induce cell death in prostate cancer cells. A study[45] revealed that genistein can induce cell death or apaptosis in prostate cancer cells revealing a dramatic reduction in PSA secretion as well as inhibiting the growth of hormone sensitive and hormone-insensitive cancer cell lines.

In preliminary results, researchers from Mount Sinai Hospital in Toronto, Ontario, Canada found that flavonoids from soy administered in vivo may significantly block PSA production. Although researchers from Wayne State University and the FDA cannot explain its mechanism of action, isoflavones seem to decrease the rate of rise in serum PSA levels while stabilizing the disease in both hormone-sensitive and refractory prostate cancers.[46] When given doses similar to those found in Asian diets, genistein had been found to reduce malignant tumors in the prostate. The isoflavones may also increase the activities of cytotoxic T cells and natural killer (NK) cells.

The compound SBA (small biologically active agent found in Haelan 951's formula) was shown to reduce prostate cancer cell size, cell growth and reduce the formation of blood vessels in prostate cancer tissue in a study on mice.[47] The results were statistically significant when compared to the control groups for the treated groups, which had a tumor inhibitory rate of more than 50 percent. This indicated that SBAs had strong antitumor effects without evidence of

---

[45] Peterson G, Barnes S., Genistein and biochanin-A inhibit the growth of human prostate cancer cell lines but not epidermal growth factor receptor tyrosine autophosphorylation. *Prostate*, 1993; 22:335-345.
[46] Colebank, Susan, "Deconstructing soy," *Health Supplement Retailer*, April, 2002.
[47] Sun F, Magna R., Hoffman R., Efficacy Evaluation of compound SBA in prostate cancer DU145 Meta Mouse Model (unpublished report, 1998, Anticancer Incorp. CA 92111

toxicity. The structural and biochemical analysis has shown that SBAs represent a group of terminally branched-chain saturated fatty acids (C 15-21) and have isolated the active anticarcinogenic ingredient as largely being contributed by 13-methyltetradecanoic acid and 12-methyl-tetradecanoic acid. Further research on these compounds have indicated that the mechanism of action of these specific branched-chain fatty acids are associated with the induction of programmed cell death (apoptosis).[48] But just as importantly it was observed that the specific branched fatty acids do not kill normal cells but inhibit the growth of cancer cells without resulting in any toxic effects.

Terminal prostate cancer

A naturopathic doctor from Portland, Oregon reported that a patient from Alabama came to him diagnosed with terminal prostate cancer. Previously, the man's oncologist had treated him with every therapy, and eventually told him, "you'd better go and get your things in order." Assuming he would die soon, the patient went out and purchased a cemetery plot, and even a gravestone. He paid for his funeral arrangements, and divested himself of most of his personal belongings. The N.D. suggested he try drinking a concentrated soybean phytochemical beverage, telling him he had nothing to lose. The man is still alive and well. When he asked the N.D. what he thought he should do with the gravestone, the doctor said, "place it in your backyard and go read it every night. It will make you feel better."

Prostate cancer with metastasis to the bone

In late 1999, Marvin had a severe case of prostate cancer with metastasis to the hipbone and spine. He could no longer walk. His wife had to carry him around, and push him in a wheelchair, an extremely difficult task for her. They moved

---

[48] Kim H, Peterson TG, Barnes S., Mechanisms of action of the soy isoflavone genistein: emerging role for its effects via transforming growth factor beta signaling pathways. *Am Jnl Clin Nut*, 1998, Dec; 68 (6): 1418S-1425S.

from their Florida home to Ohio so she could get help from their adult children. He was hospitalized twice and eventually, his condition was deemed terminal. In January 2000, his PSA count was over 200. He began taking a soybean phytochemical liquid, and by June of 2000, his PSA levels were down to 2.9. Marvin's recovery was such that he could even mop his kitchen floor by himself prior to a recent family reunion. By July of 2000, Marvin had no signs of the cancer.

Prostate cancer with lymph node infiltration
A 73 year-old gentlemen, with a PSA of 5.0 underwent tests which revealed he had prostate cancer and was scheduled for a radical prostatectomy. At the time of surgery it was discovered the cancer had spread to his lymph nodes and the lower rectal region. Surgery was performed on the lymph nodes, but not the prostate gland. Biopsies, three weeks later confirmed the cancer had spread and a course of chemotherapy and radiation was prescribed. In addition to this protocol, he took a bottle of the phytochemical beverage each day for two weeks. Several weeks later, CT scans confirmed the cancer was in remission. He continued to take a reduced protocol of the beverage and five years following his diagnosis, his blood tests came back normal and his PSA levels less than 0.1. Subsequent repeat colonoscopic examination and CT scans of the abdomen and pelvis has not revealed any evidence of metastic disease.

Squamous cell bladder & prostate cancer
On October 18 of 1999 a biopsy revealed a diagnosis of squamous cell carcinoma. Subsequent biopsies on December 3rd, 1999 and January 25, 2000 revealed the absence of a tumor. Both of these biopsies were taken and documented by Sloan Kettering Memorial Hospital. The patient, Harold Herman, was in a delicate health position. He had recently undergone surgery for a heart bypass, and brachytherapy of the prostate, along with previous radiation treatment for the prostate. Because of his age, 73, and his previous medical history, the physicians were reluctant to perform systemic

chemotherapy, or further radiation and surgery to remove the bladder. The risk of rectal injury was alarmingly high, and Mr. Herman faced having a temporary colostomy, while the surgeons tried to remove the bladder and prostate. Deciding against that surgery, Mr. Herman took himself to an alternative medicine physician in Lawrence, New York, who placed him on the following regimen:

Medications: Hytrin, Parlodal, Proscar

Supplements: multivitamin/mineral supplement, antioxidants, Vitamin C, Saw palmetto, St. John's Wort, Gingko Biloba, Genistein soy isoflavone, CoQ10, Flaxseed oil, Ther-Greens IPP, MGN-2 immune-enhancing complex, Haelan soy phytochemical concentrate (at a rate of one bottle per day).

Vaccinations: Staph, Glyoxal (homeopathic)

A biopsy performed in December 1999 showed the absence of squamous cell carcinoma in his bladder and prostate. Mr. Herman received a complete clean bill of health from all seven physicians. By the spring of 2000, Mr. Herman stated he was in remission, has energy, and recovers quickly from each cytoscopy test. He still has his bladder, exercises regularly, is cancer free according to the medical tests, and is optimistic about the future.

Use of soy with chemotherapy?

There has been a controversy for some time between those who support the use of antioxidants along with the use of chemotherapy. The original concept that antioxidants might protect cancer cells from chemotherapy came from the observation that cancer cells contained higher levels of vitamin C than normal cells. Later research showed that cancer cells did not have the enzymes necessary for the processing of vitamin C and as a result the vitamin C accumulated in the cancer cells and was in fact toxic rather than protective to the cancer cells. The ill-conceived idea that anti-oxidants might protect the cancer cells has survived extensive reports to show that cancer patients do better with antioxidant protection during chemotherapy treatments.

A study included 318 cancer patients and of those, 276 were taking chemotherapy, with the balance receiving radiation treatments in addition to consuming a fermented soy beverage. The study showed the soy protected the patients from the toxic effects of the chemotherapy with markedly reduced side effects.[49]

All cancer cells revert to a survival mechanism, known as NF-KB, within two hours of being hit with chemotherapy. A study found that cisplatin, docetaxel, and adriamycin chemotherapy agents significantly increased the cancer cell's protective NF-kB pathway activity within two hours of chemotherapy administration allowing many of the cancer cells to survive the treatments. The NF-kB inducing activity of the chemotherapeutic agents were completely abrogated in cells pre-treated with the soy isoflavone genistein producing greater apoptosis with both chemotherapy and radiation treatments. Cancer cell death in prostate, breast and pancreatic cancers as a result of pre-treatment with the soy resulted in 8-10 times greater cancer cell deaths. In this study, the results of radiation's cancer cell killing was improved by 15 percent.

Ovarian cancer and chemotherapy

A 61 year-old woman, who weighed at times up to 400 pounds, developed a mass in her abdomen. On March 15, 2001, she was diagnosed with ovarian cancer. There were several large tumors in the abdominal area with the largest being the size of a basketball and a smaller tumor the size of a softball. She was diagnosed as having terminal cancer and given only sixty days to live.

She had one round of chemotherapy in addition to drinking one bottle of the soy phytochemical beverage for twenty days. By May 15 of that year she had lost over 100

---

[49] Department of Pathology, Karmanos Cancer Institute, Wayne State University School of Medicine.

pounds and the basketball size tumor was gone. Diagnosis was that the softball sized tumor shrunk to the size of a golf ball. On further examination it was discovered that the mass was no longer a tumor, but just a pool of fluids.

Colon/rectal cancer and chemotherapy

A man had a tumor too large for surgery and received one chemotherapy treatment to shrink the tumor prior to surgery. He drank a fermented soy beverage for a short time period prior to his chemotherapy treatment. When the man went for surgery the tumor was completely gone and no surgery was performed. The surgeon stated "I've seen chemotherapy shrink the tumors a little bit but I have never seen the tumors go away completely".

Lung cancer and chemotherapy

Roxanne was an active woman, who, at the age of 46, was diagnosed with small-cell lung cancer, also known as oat cell, with lymph-node involvement. She was a heavy smoker, and had significant stress; (her cancer began after her father died, and she experienced a difficult divorce). Roxanne's doctor told her that her cancer was one of the most aggressive and fastest growing, with a life expectancy of 2-4 months. She was told that chemotherapy and radiation might extend her life for up to a year.

Her sister had heard of successes other cancer patients had experienced with a concentrated soybean drink that was produced in China. She got Roxanne to try the therapy; at first with eight ounces of this soy mixture every day. At the same time she also was receiving chemotherapy and radiation treatments. Roxanne also changed her diet to include more organic greens and fruit, and reduced her red meat intake. She altered her lifestyle to keep her stress minimal. Roxanne was part of a clinical trial group, and was told by her oncologist that she could not take the fermented soy during chemotherapy trials. Roxanne took the soy beverage anyway, and did not tell the oncologist, in order to stay in the clinical trial.

Three weeks passed after the soy therapy was started, and Roxanne was retested. The doctor expected to see a ten percent shrinkage in the tumor, a standard response to the chemotherapy, but he was surprised to find a 95 percent tumor reduction. She returned in another three weeks, and a 100 percent tumor reduction was the finding. The doctor performed bone and organ scans, and cancer growths were not detected anywhere. Roxanne's treatment plan was six 3-day series of chemotherapy (Cisplatin and VP16), along with 30 radiation treatments to the chest, and an additional 15 to her head, as this type of cancer is known to metastasize to the brain. Roxanne feels that the soybean drink made the difference. Even her doctor, who could not refute the outcome, encouraged her to continue taking it. During the chemotherapy and radiation treatments, Roxanne reported that she never got sick, or suffered the normal side effects most patients inherit. Roxanne was the only survivor in her chemotherapy clinical trial.

Other Cancers

Infant cancer
Caitlin's mother noticed a bulge in her three-month-old daughter's right eye. A doctor's visit resulted in a heart breaking diagnosis. Caitlin had a tumor surrounding her optic nerve. A week later, a further diagnosis showed three large, fast-growing cancerous tumors connecting from her eye to the base of her spine. The doctor's theory was the cancer must have developed while she was still in her mother's womb. The prognosis: she might make it to her first birthday—if she were lucky.

Caitlin was admitted into the hospital, put on IV's, and chemotherapy was started. Her mother feared this "poison," but the little girl survived the initial six months of treatment. At this time, her mother began adding, without the health provider's knowledge, some soy concentrate along with other nutrients in her bottle, and also, continued to breast-feed her when she could.

At eleven months, Caitlin began eating organic baby food, and was given Thymus Protein A and MGN3, a mushroom-based immune-system stimulant. She continued to have the soy concentrate mixed with maple syrup, and a natural banana-flavor in her baby bottle. Testing revealed that the tumors had stopped growing. They have shrunk in size and now seem to be encapsulated. Caitlin's energy is comparable with any healthy infant her age, and she even has a full head of hair and very rosy cheeks.

Skin cancer

A young boy living in Arizona was diagnosed as having a precancerous mole. With a family history of melanoma, his parents watched it closely. It eventually disappeared by itself, but his family was careful to reduce his exposure to the sun. As an adult, he again developed a skin lesion about 1/8 inch in diameter on his cheekbone. The diagnosis was cancer.

This man started drinking a soy concentrate that consisted of one 8 oz. bottle a day for the first four days, and then 1 oz. per day for the next month. The lesion shrank, so he stopped the soy and went on an internal body-cleanse. For three weeks, he consumed only alkaline foods, herbs, spirulina, and chlorella. The lesion reddened again so he returned to the soy drink. Currently, the lesion area has almost a normal skin tone. The man attributes his improvement to the soy concentrate, as he visibly saw the lesion diminish specifically during the time when he drank the soy supplement.

The National Cancer Institute has accepted the following case as "sole therapy cured" cases using Haelan's fermented soy beverage.

Liver cancer

A construction superintendent in his 60s was undergoing surgery to remove a gall-bladder blockage of his bile duct. Once they opened him up, they found that it was pinched off by cancer that had surrounded it. The doctors also found cancer in his intestines and his lymphatic system. They closed him up, with a drain to help remove the bile fluid. His cancer (cholangiocarcinoma) was so pervasive they never expected him to leave the hospital.

A friend brought him some soybean concentrate, and the man began to drink it every day for a period of two and a half weeks. After the initial two weeks, his oncologist did a fluoroscope examination, found tumor shrinkage, and ordered a CT scan to verify his findings. The man continued to drink a bottle of the Chinese soybean concentrate each day. He also took Venus flytrap, red clover, CoQ10, liquid oxygen, and pycnogenol. By the third week, the bile drain, which was supposed to drain fluid buildup, was instead being sucked back into his body. Another CT scan revealed that the liver was almost its normal size, and the drainage tube was being pulled inward. The man's initial cancer growth had been reduced by half, and the metastases in the intestines and lymphatic were gone.

Seven months later, lab reports showed that blood tests and cancer markers were near normal in all parameters with no signs of any tumors remaining. He moved after his recovery. His new doctor didn't believe he had had liver cancer, because no one is known to have survived cholangiocarcinoma. The doctor took a biopsy of the liver, comparing it with the biopsy sample from the man's initial gallbladder surgery. The test confirmed what the man had told him. The doctor was shocked that this man was alive. He did not know of any other survivors, and could not deny the man's conviction that his remission was attributed to the soy phytochemical beverage.[50]

H.I.V.- positive
In 1989, a patient tested positive for H.I.V. By June of 1990, his health had deteriorated dramatically, so much so he had the look of a full-blown AIDS patient. He had lost 30

[50] Sage, Donna, M.S.S.A., "Interview," *Townsend Letter for Doctors*, Oct. 7, 1998.

pounds, and was admitted to a Louisiana hospital for Pneumocystis Carinii Pheumonia. Death seemed imminent. His family learned of a liquid soy phytochemical concentrate, and brought it to the hospital. After several courses of the liquid concentrate, his strength and appetite returned, and soon he was released from the hospital. Three months later, after continued treatment with the soy concentrate, his weight returned to normal, his gums quit bleeding, his red blood cells increased in numbers, and he no longer needed a wheelchair. He believes the soy concentrate was the key to his much-improved health.

The following case has been submitted and accepted by the National Cancer Institute with the patient being cancer free after seven years.

Pancreatic cancer
Steve Kochak had pancreatic cancer spread throughout the intestines and gall bladder. After a protocol of several months of receiving the soy phytochemical and after having no symptoms he was tested extensively including CAT scans. These tests revealed that he was completely cancer free. The doctor who collected and verified the medical records for submittal to the National Cancer Institute as part of its best case scenario program was Vijaya Nair, M.D., M.S. Assistant Clinical Professor in Epidemiology at Columbia University, New York.

Ulna Melanoma
"At aged 25, I was diagnosed as having Rheumatoid Arthritis in 1990. My doctors prescribed *Ansaid* tablets for my condition, to relieve the pain and stiffness. Subsequently, I developed a tingling sensation in the fingers of my right hand and was diagnosed with an Ulna Melanoma tumor, visible as a lump on my right elbow. The tumor was pressing on the Ulna nerve in my right elbow, causing the sensation in my hand. The tumor was malignant, and the surgical procedure suggested was risky because of the possibility that the

nerve could be cut during the operation, leaving me little or no use of my right arm.

In April 1991, I was introduced to a liquid, soy phytochemical concentrate. I drank 8 oz. per day for two days, and then skipped two days, then repeated it for two more days. On the fifth day, I noticed that the tingling in my right-hand fingers had disappeared and it was visibly evident that the size of the tumor had decreased. By the time I visited my surgeon, the tumor was gone. Additionally, the aches and pains of my Rheumatoid Arthritis also disappeared. Fifteen of my coworkers visibly saw the tumor in my right elbow and are witness to the fact that it is now gone."
-Denis Joachim, Metairie, Louisiana

Hodgkin's lymphoma
Al was a 47 year-old family man who was stunned when he was diagnosed with Stage 4 Hodgkin's lymphoma and liver cancer. He had noticed a lump on his neck and a biopsy revealed that the growth was malignant. He underwent surgery and immediately afterwards began a protocol of the soy phytochemical beverage. Unfortunately surgery-related hepatitis had hold of him and he was so sick he discontinued the beverage. When the hepatitis subsided, doctors recommended an aggressive course of chemotherapy. Al resumed his soy beverage in conjunction with the drug therapy. He also added vitamin C, milk thistle, alpha-linolenic acid supplements, and acupuncture. But poor Al was not out of the woods.

After two chemotherapy treatments he started having major complications. The chemo had stimulated deep vein thrombosis, severe blood clotting in his right leg, which led to a 35-day hospitalization. During this time he gave up his soy beverage and was given massive doses of heparin, which he discovered he was allergic to. This caused a need for plasma transfusions because the allergy reaction was consuming his white blood cells. His leg grew worse and eventually it was amputated up to the knee. His doctors then resumed his chemotherapy. The stump of his knee became necrotic and the leg became swollen, and developed blood clots.

Al decided to again try the soy beverage internally and applied it to the black, painful knee tissue as well. To the doctors surprise the necrosis reversed. After two more chemo treatments the doctor also announced his cancer was in remission. Al notes, "My wife told the doctor it was the soy beverage and he just laughed at her and attributed this miracle to the chemotherapy." Al knew better and figured the chemo alone would have killed him.[51]

Tongue cancer
"In 1979 I was diagnosed with lesions on my tongue which persisted until 1986 when it was discovered they were malignant. The cancer had spread all through the left side of my tongue into my throat. By 1998 I was forced to undergo major surgery in addition to traditional cancer therapy. In August 2002 I began an aggressive program, which included high doses of vitamin C, an oxygenator, and the soy phytochemical. By the end of six months a visual examination revealed there was no further detection of the lesions and as of February 2003 a CT scan confirmed this. I attribute my recovery to the soy beverage, vitamin C, oxygen therapy and a lot of prayer."
-R.N., Metairie, LA.

Other Applications

World record holder
This story targets the power of immune support on our physical condition. A 74 year-old runner was a friend of Walter Wainright, a leading advocate of the concentrated soybean beverage. The man was a marathon runner, but he found that after twenty miles, he felt faint, and couldn't go on. Walter suggested he drink 4 oz. of the soybean beverage

---

[51] Sage, Donna, M.S.S.A., "Soy Nutrient Aids in Cancer Remission," *WellBeing Journal,* Jul/Aug 1999, vol 8 no. 4

before his run, and 4 oz. during. The man soon reported that not only did he run the first 20 miles, but after the second soy drink, he found that he could run an additional 20 miles.

With his improved results, he subsequently went to Plano, Texas where they log world running distance records. At the time, the record stood at 105 miles in 48 hours. The man, who was still on the soy program, ran 145 miles in 48 hours. The following year, he added another world record, running 190 miles in 72 hours. He continued taking the soy beverage. At age 79, he bested his own national 50-mile record twice, which he laughingly attributes to adding Pegasus Class II Ginsenocides to his concentrated soy drink. His body responded exceedingly well to the nutrient boost that the soy added, which exemplifies how this phytochemical beverage is not just "medicine," but shows it effectiveness as a supplement.

Laboratory Studies
In a petri dish a test was done to see if the soy phytochemical beverage could kill gastric cancer cells. The results revealed that 95, 99, and 99 percent of each test killed the cancer cells.[52]

In a controlled animal study the soy phytochemical was monitored in 130 mice that were infected with the malaria parasite. Immune system function dropped by one-third in the malaria infected group, which was receiving no treatment. In the group being administered the soy phytochemical beverage, the parasites were eliminated in 61 percent of the mice and when it was used with the Chinese malaria medication, the results proved to be 100 percent effective.[53]

Studying the somatotrophic effect of the soy beverage on dystrophic mice showed a significant improvement in

---

[52] Fujian Academy of Science, "Gastric Cancer Invivo Study," *Laboratory of tumor Research,* Nov. 30, 1991.

[53] Guangkai, Yang, Nuiwen, Ji, Jing, Wang, Cifu, Chen, Coal Miners Sanatorium of Fujian Provence, Fujian Medical College, "Effect of Haelan oral liquid on nonspecific immunity in antimalaria therapy," *Chinese Journal of Prevention of Parasite Diseases* 1990, 3(3): 240-241.

their nutritional status and growth. Dystrophy is any abnormal condition caused by defective nutrition or metabolism. The mice on the protocol were able to reach normal weight levels with the soy beverage.[54]

Summary

In the true stories you have just read, all the individuals had ingested a concentrated phytochemical soy beverage from China. The majority also changed their diets to include more fruit and vegetables, and cut back on red meat and sugar. The use of the soy concentrate lessened side effects of those patients who were undergoing chemotherapy and radiation treatments. These accounts do not surprise the Chinese, for they have used soy medicinally for over 300 years, and it has been well documented as a food staple in Asian diets for over 5,000 years.

Soy assists the body in fighting disease, and aiding the immune system by decreasing viral loads and increasing immune system functions. But, the real hero is the immune system. When it is working properly, it has the ability to know exactly how to rid the body of unwanted invaders. Unfortunately, most individuals do not support their immune system with the proper dietary tools it needs to function efficiently. In fact, many do a great deal to reduce the immune system's abilities through environmental hazards and/or lifestyle choices. Our dietary recommendations focus on two building blocks, minerals and enzymes, without which, the body will suffer and die. By reinforcing our body's natural supply of these elements, we give our immune system additional back up support, particularly when it needs to fight illness.

The liquid soybean beverage used in the studies listed in this book were manufactured by Haelan Products, Inc.

---

[54] Ziqiang, Huang, "The Somatotrophic Effect of Haelan on Dystrophic Mice," *Research and Teaching Department of Pharmacology, Fujian Medical College*, June 1, 1993.

During the past ten years, the company has amassed a list of over 6,000 professional health care workers who recommend the product for cancer patients and those suffering from immune system related health problems. There are more than ten hospitals that have performed various animal and human trials using their fermented soy formulation and these studies include various types of human cancers in animal models.

The Haelen has been found to be anti-viral, anti-inflammatory, anti-allergy, anti-cancer, and a vasodilator, The anti-viral capability of the Haelan is a big benefit to the immune system, because it is able to kill viral infections that are too tough for the immune system to handle alone. An NCI study showed that the soybean "BB" saponins stop the replication of HIV. Users of the soybean beverage also report Hepatitis- C viral load decreased quite rapidly.

These studies are available in the United States upon request from U.S. Research Reports, Inc. Index of Studies. Contact number: (800) 533-9660.

7

Striving for Disarmament

Soy, as we have stated in the chapters previously, is extremely beneficial. Consumed on a daily basis, it will add tremendous support to the immune system. Medicinally, soy's effectiveness is enhanced through a specific process that allows the nutrients to pass into the cell, even through the thick walls of cancer cells. You might want to understand what makes the soybean concentrate from China, mentioned in our success stories, so powerful a healing modality for all those patients. The answer is two-fold; naturally occurring phytochemicals (researchers have discovered over 103,000 of them), and the specialty processing of soybeans that allow entry of these nutrients into the cancer cell itself.

Phytochemicals, as mentioned previously, are anti-inflammatory, antibacterial, antiviral, antiosteoporotic, anti-mutagenic, antiarcinogenic and capture free-radicals, preventing them from damaging DNA. They have been shown to reduce the incidence of breast cancer, prostate, and colon cancers along with lowering cholesterol, detoxifying the liver, clearing up bronchitis, alleviating pain, treating stomach ulcers, and stopping cramps.

The benefits of soy, especially the advantage we receive from isoflavones, can be crucial to disarming cancer. Reports show that 25-50 percent of hospital cancer patients suffer from Protein Calorie Malnutrition and only 1/3 of them survive five years. Chemotherapy and radiation are sufficient stressors to induce Protein Calorie Malnutrition in a patient.[55] Also, taking one tablespoon per day of a soybean food concentrate as a preventive medicine adds 50-80 mg. of isoflavones, such as genistein, in the diet. This level is extremely hard to achieve just by eating soy foods. For

---

[55] Block, K.I., M.D., "The effects of diet on quality and quantity of life in cancer patients, symposium," *Adjuvant Nutrition for Cancer Patients*, Nov 6, 1992, Tulsa, OK.

example, the soy food with the highest concentration of Genistein is soy miso. It takes approximately 2000 grams (714 ounces) per day, of the fermented soy food miso to achieve equal levels of genistein, as stated above. As a source of protein, soy requires a lower amount of energy for the kidneys to filter waste compared to the stress that meat and other protein foods place on them. The Chinese have used soy to treat kidney disease for more than 1,000 years. There are clinical trials and research from Japan that support the benefits of soy to treat kidney diseased patients in hospitals. This is extremely important when the body needs to fight disease around the clock.

To make a medicinal soy liquid that has an effective potency several steps are taken. Through the fermentation process, the starches and sugars are eliminated, which produces a concentration of the phytochemicals and proteins. This hydrolyzed soy protein liquid becomes a free-form amino acid, which has been found to enter the bloodstream effectively. The soy liquid protein levels have achieved blood protein levels of up to 8½ percent, comparable to hospital treatments administered through an I.V., which averaged results between 8-11 percent. This is an especially important factor to underscore for protein deficient cancer patients. Soy's benefits for the immune system are profound in the manner in which penetration is accomplished into the cancer cell, where its constituents can effectively weaken it. One company's[56] processing breaks down the naturally occurring isoflavones, from 500-3,000 daltons to 200 daltons in size. These are referred to as Small Biologically Active Isoflavones (SBAIs) which are small enough to successfully penetrate the cell wall. The nitrogenation process connects high levels of nitrogen atoms, usable to the body, directly to the small bioactive isoflavone.

The fermentation process hydrolyzes many of these soybean proteins into bioactive amino acids and compounds, consisting of various fermentation metabolites of the

---

[56] Haelan Products, Inc., Woodinville, WA .

naturally occurring isoflavones, protease inhibitors, saponins, phytosterols, and phytic-acids compounds. This nitrogenated compound is readily absorbed by the cancer cell, and provides a camouflaged entry for the anticancer proteins and phytochemicals. Once inside, the soybean protein isolate destroys blood vessels by changing the DNA back to normal. This reprogramming shuts off the release of the enzyme that dissolves blood capillaries and promotes angiogenesis (the production of new blood vessels) that feed tumor growth. Once the cancer cell is disabled and weakened, the immune system and the T-cells can use the nitric acid to dissolve them. *It is this process that makes specific concentrated, soybean liquids so distinctive.*

The primary soybean isoflavone that most effectively inhibits cancer cellular growth, is genistein.[57] The National Cancer Institute in Bethesda, Maryland, has identified and written on the results of genistein ingestion. Genistein has inhibited cell growth in skin cancer, leukemia, lung cancer, prostate, colon, precolon, and breast cancer.[58] The National Cancer Institute researchers at the University of Southern California in Los Angeles, through animal testing programs, identified genistein-stopping cells from making the stress proteins that are produced by cancer cells. Those proteins help cancer cells survive attacks by the body's immune system, and anticancer therapies. Physicians in the U.S. and Mexico are using the extracted genistein against many forms of cancers. They are reporting positive results against many forms of cancers.

In addition to cancer research, the soy concentrate continues to be tested for other benefits. One example is a clinical study that was conducted over a four-month period, involving 303 healthy persons aged 50-69, with no apparent problems with their livers, kidneys, or any other health issues. The study results showed that nitrogenated, liquid,

[57]Ogawara, H., et al., "A specific inhibitor for tyrosine protein kinase from pseudomonas," *Journal Antibiotics*, 1985.
[58] Bowen, R., et al, " Antipromotional effect of the soybean isoflavone genistein," *Proc. American Assn. Cancer Research*, 1993.

highly concentrated soybean beverage seems to reverse the aging process and improve the overall health of this test group.

The study's documented results are as follows:

▶ Increases brain function;
▶ Increases immune CD3 and CD4 cells;
▶ Increases the production of interferons and interlukens;
▶ Increases volumetric lung function approximately 25 percent;
▶ Increases the cytotoxic effects of the NK killer immune cells;
▶ Increases volumetric pumping capacity of the heart by 25 percent;
▶ Balances levels of testosterone and estriol sex hormones in men and women;
▶ Increases cellular levels of zinc, copper, manganese, and superoxide-dismutase antioxidant enzymes.

It is important to note that a liquid soybean concentrate has been a parallel therapy in many of the documented cases, alongside traditional cancer treatments, such as chemotherapy and radiation. The soy benefits are strengthening of the immune system and a reduction in side effects normally associated with these types of treatments.

The concentrate also has been documented in the treatment of other types of illnesses, such as Parkinson's, Muscular Dystrophy, viral infections, gangrene, and hepatitis. It also has been used as an adjunct treatment for Alzheimers-like dementia because it seems to "recharge" inactive neurons in the brains.[59] As a brain target, where mineral deficiencies tend to impair function, the soy concentrate is extremely beneficial, especially when used in conjunction with a crystalloid electrolyte formula. Mental acuity with soy

---

[59] Walker, M., D.P.M., "Concentrated soybean phytochemicals," *Healthy & Natural magazine,* vol 2, no. 2, April 1995.

therapy has shown improvement. Additionally, the saponins in soy have inhibitory effects against the infectivity of the human immunodeficiency virus (HIV), associated with AIDS.

Soy alone should not be viewed as a singular cancer-cure. It is an adjuvant (helpful) nutrition in cancer treatments. Results from nutritional boosters, such as soy,[60] indicate a reduced toxicity of chemotherapy on the patient, and enhanced toxicity on tumor cells. Nutritional boosters also treat malnutrition from cachexia (wasting), anorexia, and parasitic tumors, stimulate the immune system into above-normal activity, protect against carcinogenic treatment, and reduce vulnerability to long-term effects of cancer treatment.

Clinical evidence also indicates that selective nutrition may be able to influence the cancer process even after initiation. Although adjuvant nutrition is not encouraged or endorsed as the sole therapy for aggressive cancer, it may prevent Protein Calorie Malnutrition, which has been linked to increased mortality, surgical failures, reduced response to chemotherapy, slow wound-healing, weakness, and apathy. In the Journal of Orthomolecular Medicine, a study followed 129 diagnosed cancer patients for eleven years while they were being treated with traditional oncology methods. Of those patients, 31 nutritionally untreated patients' life spans averaged less than 6 months and those whose treatments included adjuvant nutrition programs, experienced a 75-2100 percent improvement in life-spans.[61]

Food guidelines offered in the same research report advised eating less animal fats and sugar, and replacing animal protein with vegetable proteins. Animal fats are conducive to the body's production of arachidonic acid and prostaglandin 2, which amplifies immunosuppression and promotes tumor growth. Omega-3 fatty acids (from flax and fish oil), help in reducing the production of arachidonic acid, and

---

[60] "U.S. Research Reports, Inc., Report No. 100," Metairie, LA, January 15, 1993. (800) 533-9660.

[61] Hoeffer, A., Pauling, L., "Mortality Data of Cancer Patients," *Journal of Orthmolecular Medicine*, vol 5 no. 3, 1990.

produces an environment in the body which is not conducive to tumor growth or metastasis.[62]

The report also encouraged high-fiber grains and cereals. The active ingredient in fiber is the phytic-acid compound that causes the inner lining of the colon to slough off remaining poisons and toxins embedded in the colon wall. This ingredient is far more important in maintaining health of the colon, than the fibers themselves. Also found in high-fiber foods is an anticancer micronutrient, inositiol hexa-phosphate. Vegetables and soy were highlighted, as they contain isoflavones, protease inhibitors, saponins, phytosterols, and inositol hexaphosphate, the anticancer micronutrient also found in fiber.

People with cancer can become malnourished because of negative influences due to hospitalization, radiation, chemotherapy, pre-existing conditions such as smoking, alcohol abuse, poor dietary habits, malabsorption syndromes, food sensitivities, or immunological stress. Max Gerson, M.D., in his book, *A Cancer Therapy* indicated that cancer is caused by nutrient deficiency and cellular toxicity.[63] Along with proper nutritional habits that incorporate soy, (especially fermented and nitrogenated soy formulas), individuals can overturn disease-preying deficiencies, and become closer to disarming cancer.

---

[62] Blackburn, G., M.D., Ph.D., in Symposium Adjuvant Nutrition for Cancer Patients, 1992.
[63] Gerson, Max, M.D., *A Cancer Therapy, 5th Edition,* The Talman Press, 57.

Resources:

-Haelan, Inc., Soy Health Products.
Fermented soybean, oral-nutritional beverages that are manufactured with Nitrogenation process, grown organically in mineral-rich soil and harvested at peak phytochemical production.
18568 142nd Ave. NE, Woodinville, WA 98072
(800) 542-3526 www.haelan951.com

-Nature's Path, Inc.
Liquid, crystalloid electrolyte mineral supplement.
P.O. Box 7862, Venice, FL 34287
(800) 326-5772 www.naturespathinc.com

-LJB Piper, LLC
electroBlast™ effervescent electrolyte tablets with no sugar or artificial sweeteners. Dissolves in water to make a refreshing lemon-lime drink.
P.O. Box 1454, Lakeville, CT 06039
(888) 217 7233 www.electroblast.com

-Prozyme Products, Inc.
Organic digestive enzymes for people and animals.
6444 N. Ridgeway Ave., Lincolnwood, IL 60712
(800) 252-5537 www.prozyme.net

-Sedna Specialty Health Products
Sprouted soy powder supplement, dried at low temperatures to maintain maximum nutrient levels.
P.O. Box 606, Hendersonville, NC 28793
(800) 223-0858

-Carico International
Multi-stage water filers with submicron ceramic adsorbents to address all priority pollutants including micro-organisms.
P.O. Box 60052, Staten Island, NY 10306
(888) 424-7873 or (718) 667-7022   www.carico.com

INDEX

Bibliography

-Anderson, Nina & Dr. Howard Peiper, *Crystalloid Electrolytes,* Safe Goods, CT, 1998.

-Anderson, Nina & Dr. Howard Peiper, *The All-Natural High Performance Diet,* Safe Goods, CT, 1999.

-Anderson, Nina & Dr. Howard Peiper, *The Secrets of Staying Young,* Safe Goods, CT, 1998.

-Blackburn,G., M.D., Ph.D., *Advanced Cancer: A New Challenge in Nutritional Medicine,* Symposium Adjuvant Nutrition for Cancer Patients, Nov. 6, 1992

-Bowen, R., Barnes S., Wei, H., "Antipromotional effect of the soybean isoflavone genistein," *Proc. American Assn. Cancer Research,* 34-555, Abstract 3310, 1993.

-Colebank, Susan, "Deconstructing Soy," *Health Supplement Retailer,* April 2002.

-Crook, Thomas H., Ph.D. and Brenda Adderly, M.H.A., *The Memory Cure,* Pocket Books, New York, 1998.

-Divi, R.L., Chang, H.C., "Anti-thyroid isolfavones from soybean: isolation, characterization, and mechanisms of action, *Biochem Pharmacol,* 1997, Nov. 15; 54 (10):1087-96.

-Fujian Academy of Science, "Gastric Cancer Invivo Study," *Laboratory of tumor Research,* Nov. 30, 1991.

-Gerson, Max, M.D., "Gastric Cancer Invivo Study," Laboratory of Tumor Research, Fujian Academy of Science, November 20, 1991-, *A Cancer Therapy,* 5th Edition, The Talman Press, 57.

-Gotoh T., Yamada, K., Ito, A., Yin, H., Kataoka, T., Dohi, K., "Chemoprevention of N-nitroso-N-metylurea-induced rat mammary cancer by miso and tamoxifen, alone and in combination," *Jpn J Cancer Res,* 1998; 89:487-95.

-Goyoh, T., Yamada, K., Yin, H., Ito, A., Kataoka, T., Dohi, K., "Chemoprevention of N-nitroso-N-methylurea-induced rat mammary carcinogenesis by soy foods or biochanin," A. Jpn," *J Cancer Res,* 1998; 89: 137-42.

-Grant, J.P., "Proper use and recognized role of total parenteral nutrition in the cancer patient," *Nutrition,* vol 6, no. 4 July/Aug 1990.

-Grun, I.U., Adhikari, K., Li C, et al., "Changes in the profile of genistein, daidzein and their conjugates during thermal processing of tofu," *J Agric Food Chem,* June 2001; 49(6):2839-43.

-Hartley, Bonnie, "Is Soy a Ploy," *Healthy & Natural Journal,* vol 4, issue 2 38-40.

-Hoeffer, A., Pauling, L., *Mortality Data of Cancer Patients,"* Journal of Orthmolecular Medicine, vol 5, no 3, 143, 1990.

-Holt, Steven, M.D., *Soya for Health: The Definitive Medical Guide,* 1996, Mary Ann Liebert, Inc.

-Huang Ziqiang, "The Somatotrophic Effect of Haelan on Dystrophic Mice," *Research and Teaching Department of Pharmacology, Fujian Medical College,* June 1, 1993.

-Kennedy, A.R., Billings, P.C., *Anticarcinogenic actions of protease inhibitors.*

Anticarcinogenesis and Radiation Protection, Plenum, N.Y., 285-295, 1987.

-Kennedy, A.R., "The conditions for the modification of radiation transformation in vitro by a tumor promoter and protease inhibitors," *Carcinogenesis,* 6: 1441-1445, 1985.

-Lazennec, G., Bresson, D., Lucas, A., Chauveau, C., Vignon, F., "ER Beta Inhibits Proliferation and Invasion of Breast Cancer Cells," Endocrinology, 2001: 142:4120-30.

-Mason, Roger, *No More Horse Estrogen,* Safe Goods, 2001

-Messina ,M., Barnes, S., "The Role of Soy Products in Reducing Risk of Cancer," J Natl Cancer Inst, 1991, 83, 541-546.

-Morabia, A. Costanza, M.C., "International variability in ages at menarche, first live birth and menopause, World Health Organization Collaborative Study of Neoplasia and Steroid Contraceptives," [published erratum appears in Am J Epidemiol, Sept 1999; 150(5):546], *Am J Epidemiol,* 1998, 148:1195-205.

-Nair, Vijaya, M.D., M.S., and Vic Hernandez, M.P.H., "A novel Fermented Soya Beverage and Safe Nutritive Adjunct in Prostate Cancer Therapies: Is There a Possible Chemopreventive Role?, *Townsend Letter for Doctors & Patients,* July. 2002.

-Ogawara, H., Akiyama, T., Isbida, J., Watanabe, S., Suzuki, K., "A specific inhibitor for tyrosine protein kinase from pseudomonas", *Journal Antiobiotics,* 39: 606-608, 1985.

-Peterson, G., Barnes, S., "Genistein Inhibition of The Growth of Human Breast Cancer Cells; Independence from Estrogen Receptors. The Multi-Drug Resistance Gene," Biochem Biophys Res Commun 1991; 179:661-7.

-Peterson, G., Barnes, S., "Genistein Inhibits Both Estrogen and Growth Factor-Stimulated Proliferation of Human Breast Cancer Cells." Cell Growth Differ, 1996;7:1345-51.

-Rose, D.P., Boyar, A. P., Wynder, E.L., "International comparison of mortality rates for the cancer of the breast, ovary, prostate and colon, and per capita food consumption," *Cancer,* 1986: 58: 2363-2371.

-Sage, Donna, M.S.S.A. "Soy Nutrient Gives New Hope to Cancer Patients," *WellBeing Journal,* March/April 1999.

-Sage, Donna, "Haelan Fermented Soy Product Nutritional Supplementation for the Cancer Patient," *Townsend Letter for Doctors & Patients,* October, 1998.

-Sage, Donna, M.S.S.A., "Healing Lung Cancer with Soy Nutrients," *WellBeing Journal,* May/June 1999.

-Shao, A.M., Wu, J., Shen, Z.Z., Barsky, S.H., "Genistein Exerts Multiple Suppressive Effects on Human Breast Carcinoma Cells," Cancer Res 1998L 58:4851-7.

-Shu, X.O, Jin, F., Qu, D., et al. "Adolescent soy food intake and other dietary habits," *Proc Am Assoc Cancer Res,* 2000; 41:94 (abstract 602).

-Soyfoods and Cancer http://www.talksoy.com

-Steinberg, Phillip N., *Isoflavones and the New Concentrated Soy Supplements,* Healing Wisdom Publications, N.Y., 1996.

-Stephens, F.O., "Phytoestrogens and prostate cancer: possible preventive role,"

Medical J Aust, 1997, 167:138-140.

-U.S. Research Reports, Inc. Report No. 107, 1996, Metarie, LA.

-Tikkanen, M.J., Wahala,K., Ojala, S., Vibrna, V. Aldercreutz, H., 1995, In 68th Scientific Sessions of the American Heart Assn. Abstract.

-Wainright, Walter, *Man to Man Meeting*, American Cancer Society presention (video), June 24, 1999.

-Walker, Morton, D.P.M., "Concentrated soybean phytochemicals," *Healthy & Natural*, vol 2, no. 2, April 1995.

-Walker, Morton, D.P.M., *The Soybean Concentrate from China for Reversing Metastatic Cancer*, Explore, vol 7, no. 2, 1996.

-White, Lon R., M.D., M.P.II, Petrovitch, Ilclcn, M.D., ct al; *Brain Aging and Midlife Tofu Consumption*, National Institute on Aging, University of Hawaii at Manoa from www.am-coll-nutr.org/jacn/vol_19/no_2/ 242.

-"WHO issues New Healthy Life Expectancy Rankings," *Press release*, World Health Organization 2000, June 2000, Washington D.C. and Geneva, Switzerland.

-Wilmore, D.W., "Catabolic Illness, Strategies for enhancing recovery," *England Journal Medicine*, vol. 325, no. 10, 695, Sept. 1991.

-Yang, Guangkai, Ji, Nuiwen, Wang, Jing, Chen, Cifu, Coal Miners Sanitorium of Fujian Provence, Fujian Medical college, "Effect of Haelan oral liquid on nonspecific immunity in antimalaria therapy," *Chinese Journal of Prevention of Parasite Diseases* 1990, 3(3): 240-241.

-Zhou J.R., "Prevention of Orthotropic Growth of Estrogen-Dependent Human Breast Tumor In Mice by Dietary Soy Phytochemicals," 222nd American Chemical Society Meeting. Chicago, Illinois 2001: Abstract 121.

-Ziqiang, Huang, "Lowering Toxic Effects of Chemotherapy & Radiation," *Research and Teaching Dept. of Pharmacology*, Fujian Medical College, Fuzhou, Peoples Republic of China, January 16, 1992.

-Ziqiang, Huang, "Protecting the Liver," *Research & Teaching Dept. of Pharmacology*, Fujian Medical College, Fuzhou, Peoples Republic of China, January 16, 1992.

The ADD and ADHD Diet	$ 9.95 US
	$14.95 CN
ADD, The Natural Approach	$ 4.95 US
	$ 6.95 CN
Testosterone is your Friend	$ 8.95 US
	$12.95 C
Eye Care Naturally	$ 8.95 US
	$12.95 CN
The Natural Prostate Cure	$ 6.95 US
	$10.95 CN
Macrobiotics for Americans	$ 7.95 US
	$11.95 CN
Minerals You Need	$ 4.95 US
	$ 6.95 CN
What is Beta Glucan	$ 4.95 US
	$ 6.95 CN
Overcoming Senior Moments	$ 7.95 US
	$11.95 CN
No More Horse Estrogen	$ 7.95 US
	$11.95 CN
Live Disease Free	$ 9.95 US
	$14.95 CN
The Secrets of Staying Young	$ 9.95 US
	$14.95 CN
Atlantis Today – The USA	$ 9.95 US
	$14.95 CN
2012 Airborne Prophesy	$16.95 US
	$24.95 CN
Analyzing Sports Drinks	$ 4.95 US
	$ 6.95 CN

For a complete listing of books visit our web site:
www.safegoodspub.com to order or call (888) 628-8731
for a free catalog (888) NATURE-1